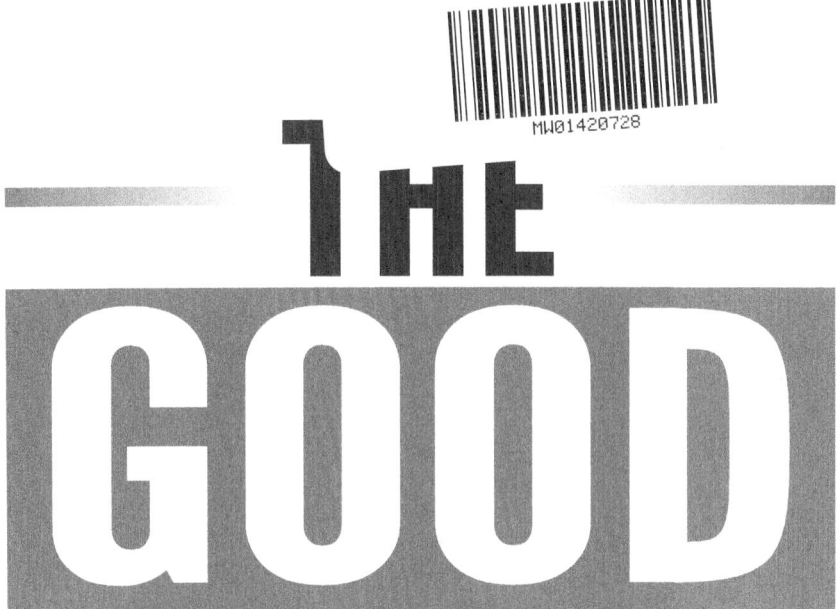

THE GOOD DOCTOR

*Motivated by a passion
for caring and health*

J. E. Block, MD, PhD, FACP

The Good Doctor
© 2015 by J. E. Block, MD, PhD, FACP

All rights reserved. No part of this book may be reproduced or transmitted in any form or by any means, electronic or mechanical, including photocopying and recording, or by an information storage and retrieval system, without permission in writing from the author.

Scripture quotation marked "NIV" is taken from the *Holy Bible, New International Version®*, NIV® Copyright ©1973, 1978, 1984, 2011 by Biblica, Inc.® Used by permission. All rights reserved worldwide.

Scripture quotation marked "NABRE" is taken from the *New American Bible, revised edition* © 2010, 1991, 1986, 1970. Confraternity of Christian Doctrine, Inc., Washington, DC. Used by permission. All rights reserved.

Cover image, Master Classic II Stethoscope, permission provided by 3M.

All stories related in this book are based on actual events, but some names have been changed or left out to maintain confidentiality for those involved.

ISBN: 978-1-943361-04-5
E-book ISBN: 978-1-943361-05-2

Library of Congress Control Number: 2015949744

Printed in the United States of America.

CONTENTS

INTRODUCTION..5
CHAPTER ONE: DOOMED FOR SUCCESS.......................7
CHAPTER TWO: BORN TO BE A DOCTOR......................13
CHAPTER THREE: A FATHER'S INFLUENCE.................25
CHAPTER FOUR: THE SCHOOL YEARS...........................35
CHAPTER FIVE: THE INTEGRATIVE APPROACH........51
CHAPTER SIX: THIS I BELIEVE...57
CHAPTER SEVEN:
AN AFFAIR OF THE HEART:
THE JOHN TAYLOR STORY...63
CHAPTER EIGHT:
A DESCENT INTO DARKNESS: KAYE'S STORY.............73
CHAPTER NINE: MEDICAL SCHOOL.................................87
CHAPTER TEN:
COMPOUNDING ISSUES: CRYSTAL'S STORY.................97
CHAPTER ELEVEN: A ROSE BY ANY
OTHER NAME IS STILL A ROSE: ROSE'S STORY........105
CHAPTER TWELVE: IS IT WORTH DYING FOR?........117
CHAPTER THIRTEEN:
DON'T WORRY! BE HAPPY!..131
CHAPTER FOURTEEN:
MARRIED TO MEDICINE..141
CHAPTER FIFTEEN: ON TO MISSOURI.........................157

CHAPTER SIXTEEN: THE NODES HAVE IT:
THE JOHN CASTRO STORY...........165

CHAPTER SEVENTEEN:
SERIOUS SINUSES: CAROL'S STORY...........177

CHAPTER EIGHTEEN: MY SPIRITUAL JOURNEY......191

CHAPTER NINETEEN:
SPIRITUAL LESSONS LEARNED...........201

CHAPTER TWENTY:
OUR UNWRITTEN STORY...........213

INTRODUCTION

Good.

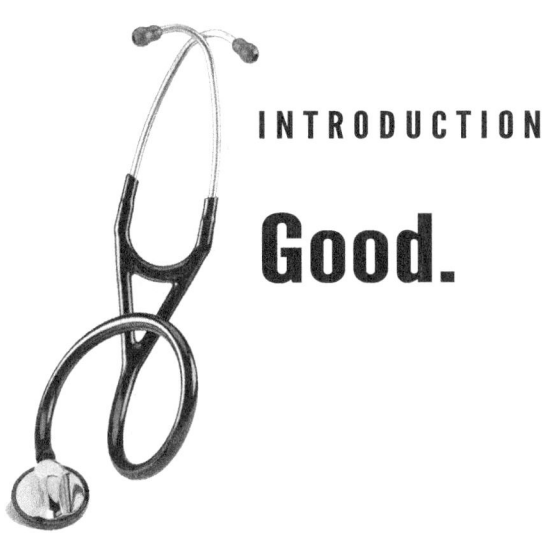

I like that word. Good conveys quality without all the hype that words like Amazing! Great! and Awesome! have always carried with them. It seems that we're bombarded with that kind of hyperbole every day. But Good is simple. It's a refreshing change of pace.

The dictionary puts the word "good" in the same category with Virtuous, Righteous, and Excellent.

Wow. That's a pretty high standard to live up to. Am I a good man? I don't know…I suppose I have my days. I just hope that at the end of my days on this planet, that my life will be judged as good.

But one thing I believe with all my heart; after a lifelong pursuit of medicine, I know I can call my practice "Good." And that's not just me talking. It's born out by the tens of thousands of patients I've seen over the years.

The Good Doctor

To me, a Good Doctor is a physician committed to practicing Good Medicine. And what is good medicine? Good medicine can be traditional or alternative, practiced by a MD or a DO, a chiropractor, a RN, an acupuncturist, naturopath, aroma therapist or masseuse.

You see, I believe good medicine is medicine focused on the patient, on her needs, his hurts, aches, pains, and disease. That may sound obvious and I suppose it should be. I've spent a lifetime battling approaches to medicine that are about almost anything but the patient. So many medical practices today focus much more on the tests, the reports, and the probabilities, than the poor, ailing patient sitting in the exam room. Even worse, modern medicine has become about the technology, the pharmacology, and the threat of malpractice litigation. It's a shame but many doctors are motivated, not by their care and compassion for the patient, but by their own agendas, whatever they may be. Those are not good doctors in my book.

Good medicine does whatever it takes to find the answer for the patient, no matter which quarter of the medical community that answer might come from. To me, it's simple; a good doctor is someone who practices good medicine.

Through all my years of school and the decades of practice and the thousands and thousands of patients I've seen over the years, I've always only wanted one thing...

to be a good doctor.

"The art is long, life is short, opportunity fleeting, experiment dangerous, judgment difficult." -Hippocrates

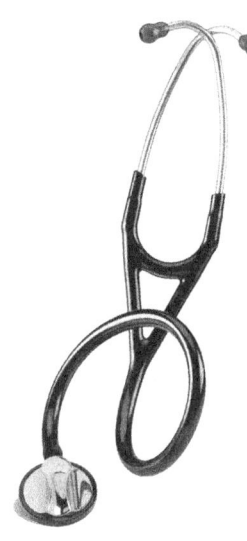

CHAPTER ONE:

DOOMED FOR SUCCESS

The darkness was complete save the thin slit of hallway light spilling into the space underneath the closet door. As he looked around through the dim light, the three year old boy could just make out the jumble of odds and ends cluttering the tiny recess. Exposed to the full light of day, there would be nothing scary in the space, just a few brooms and mops, boxes, assorted tools and other household clutter thrown in helter-skelter. But in the mind and imagination of the little boy, the wan light cast evil shadows across his mind. To him, the small place was wicked and full of harmful intent.

The boy had been grabbed by the shoulders and shoved into the closet like so much-discarded junk. The closet doorway was low and the mother had to duck to keep from hitting her head. The boy lost his balance and stumbled over a broom handle and fell with his face to the dusty floor. By the time he regained his feet, the door had slammed shut and the bolt had slid into place with deafening finality. The small boy

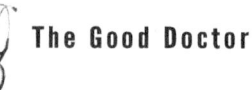 **The Good Doctor**

thought he was going to die. What made it even worse was that it was his mother who had locked him away in this prison under the stairs.

The punishment was cruel to be sure; to be thrown in the storage closet by his own mother released deep-seated demons in the mind of the young boy. The closet darkness surrounded him and began to slide its inky fingers around his chest and squeeze him tight in an unbearable embrace of terror.

He tried to scream. But the fear and the dust from the closet combined to make crying out impossible. Never mind the fact that the only one to cry out to was his mother and she was the one who had locked him in the closet in the first place.

He fell to the dirty floor and sobbed. He could still overhear his mother's shrieks as she ranted throughout the house. The boy was scared and confused. He was alone and the darkness was closing in. He heard his mother's footsteps coming closer...

Truly this is a frightening story. But to me, it's more than just a story. It was my life.

I was that boy in the closet.

It would be a tragic story if it only happened once. But incidents like this had become a regular occurrence. I was probably whining about something...the details are lost to time. But I was unhappy and I was letting my mother know, in no uncertain terms, just how unhappy I was. She finally snapped and lashed out at me, yelling, "I'll take care of you!" She grabbed me by the shoulders and shoved me into the closet under the stairs.

DOOMED FOR SUCCESS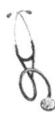

Just a few months after being locked in the closet I was bound with a clothesline from my ankles to my neck because I had displeased my mother in some way.

I still remember lying bound on the living room floor unable to move. In those days, a cheap way to cover the floors was with linoleum that mimicked the look of the carpet. I can still see that cheap floor covering in my mind's eye all these years later.

My mother was lost in her rage as she bound the clothesline cord tightly around my ankles. She continued to wrap the cord around my body, like a mummy's wrap, all the way up to my neck, my arms bound snug to my sides. Once she reached my shoulders, she wrapped the remaining cord around my small neck. Around and around. In a final act of unbelievable cruelty, she took hold of the leftover cord and pulled with all her might trying to strangle me. I was certain I was going to die. Then, when she felt she wasn't able to get the cord tight enough, she used her own hands to choke me to death. I can still feel the constriction around my neck and my Adam's apple beginning to crush.

But as quickly as it began, it faded away. Inexplicably my mother's anger started to seep out of her and she gradually let go. With no explanation or apology, she simply got up off the floor and walked away without a word. Without her holding onto the rope, it began to fall away and I was able to escape. But the effects of that incident continued to haunt me. Looking back, it's easy to see that my mother's erratic behavior was getting worse. Being thrown in a closet is a terrible thing to do to a child but it's passive in nature. Being bound with clothesline and strangled is a violent action. Her episodes were clearly escalating.

The Good Doctor

I know now that my mother was suffering from the same thing I see so often in my practice. She was struggling to deal with her post-partum depression brought about by not enough progesterone in her body following my delivery. After my birth, my mother's mental state had descended into darkness. She had become unpredictable and erratic. She was prone to fits of anger and most of the time that anger was directed towards me. Her behavior caused a deepening depression. She was ultimately institutionalized at the Philadelphia State Hospital at Byberry.

In these days of enlightenment about such things, it's hard to imagine a place more grim and depressing as Byberry. The place was crammed to overflowing with patients who struggled with everything from rather simple mental challenges to the criminally insane. Patients were forced to sleep in the hallways when the hospital exceeded capacity. Many of these same hallways were lined with raw sewage. The patients were routinely abused and taken advantage of. It's incredible to imagine that this is the environment where my mother was sent to get over her depression. It's a miracle she got better at all.

ASHES TO GOLD

At the time, my mother truly did intend to harm me. I felt the effects of violence! I experienced abandonment and betrayal by my very own mother! Sadly, many people with similar childhood nightmares have been harmed for a lifetime. They have never been able to get over the terrible things done to them when they were children. Deep-seated fear, abandonment, betrayal, and injury continue to haunt them and affect their decisions and relationships long into adulthood.

DOOMED FOR SUCCESS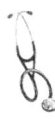

To be sure, I was shaped by those horrific childhood experiences. But God has allowed them to become the very source of my compassion toward my patients. When I walk into a consultation room and see a patient who is alone or feels abandoned, it awakens something deep inside me. When I talk to a patient who is bound up in terror because of the unknown thing happening in their body, I can't help but reach out. These people are suffering as I suffered and it's because of that suffering that I have an extra gear of compassion for my patients. Thank God that what the enemy meant for harm in my life has turned out to be the very source of my passion for medicine and compassion for my patients. I'm also thankful for the examples set before me in my early training. They showed me genuine humanity and its importance in health care.

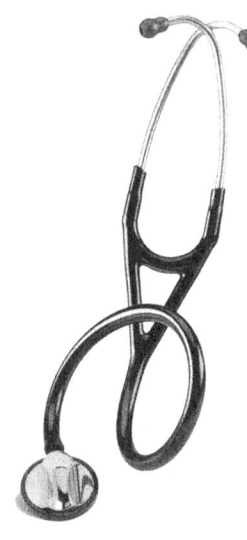

CHAPTER TWO:

BORN TO BE A DOCTOR

I believe that innovating people, called eccentric by some, are born that way.

It is not nature versus nurture, but rather a genetic designation along with the superimposition of the tribulations of life that decide our fate. Genetics point the gun, but it's Environment that pulls the trigger. This is true of you and me and the thousands of people we touch throughout our lives either physically or vicariously.

In the case of this physician, it is both! It is a true statement that good doctors are born, not made. Good doctors are honed in life's hot crucible of molding and refining, just like I was.

I don't just think this is true. I'm convinced it is.

I've seen way too many bad doctors in my lifetime to believe otherwise. Medical schools do their level best to graduate quality physicians every single year. They may walk across the stage, shake hands with the Dean and earn their degrees, but many of these people are not good doctors in my

The Good Doctor

book. Good doctors possess much more than just head knowledge of how to practice medicine. There's something far deeper, far more mysterious and powerful at work. You may not quite be able to put your finger on it, but you know it when you see it. They have the soul of a physician.

And that's something that can only be embedded into your DNA at birth. That's why good doctors are born, not made!

Sure, you can go to school to learn the science. You can even put on the white coat and wear the stethoscope around your neck. You can spend years as an intern and resident to learn the best medical practices. You can spend years as an intern, later a resident, and even obtain an advance fellowship in a medical specialty to learn the best medical science and practice. You can sit through hours of lectures and stay awake for days working in a teaching hospital. You can see hundreds of patients a week in a vibrant practice. You can lecture, even publish articles in the leading medical journals, and impress your colleagues with the depth of your knowledge and insight.

But these things alone will never give you the real human soul of a doctor. Lectures and white coats will never connect you to the hearts of your patients. Science and study can never pull empathy and compassion out of your belly. They can't teach you how to really care for your patients beyond their affliction or disease. Most doctors treat the *disease in the patient* rather than the *patient with the disease*. That caring, that soul, has to come from your gut, from that place deep inside; it's the spirit that drives everything else you do. You've either been born with it or you haven't.

Not only was I born with it, but I've been consumed by it since I was a young boy. And over the years, I've sacrificed and been punished and scarred deeply by it.

BORN TO BE A DOCTOR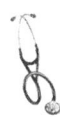

It's simple really. I was born to be a doctor. Being a doctor is part of the fabric of who I am; it's woven into the magnificent tapestry that my life has become. For as long as I can remember, I never wanted to be anything else. When other boys my age were dreaming of becoming a fireman or a movie star or even the starting shortstop for the New York Yankees, I could only think about being a doctor. Since I made up my mind, nothing has been able to distract me from this lifetime pursuit.

AN EARLY FOCUS

Over the years, I've had plenty of opportunities to give up. Early on, I wasn't an especially good student. I lacked the focus necessary to do well in the classroom.

In those days educators didn't know what to do with students like me. I was simply classified as a dumb boy with a tendency to get into trouble. This was decades before the diagnosis of ADD or, in my case ADHD, was even considered, let alone diagnosed. Even the fact that I was held back in the fifth grade ultimately contoured my future life.

I was not to be deterred. Success in the classroom came later to me. I was accepted into college but only on probation because of my low grades in high school. I had to learn quickly how to study and would stay up late into the night. I would get up early to study before school started. It's become a lifelong habit for me to rise in the middle of the night to study and later, to read medical journals and my own published writings. I typically get up for a few hours to read before going back to bed briefly, getting up in time for school, work, or even play.

The Good Doctor

I've learned that what I've done most of my life is actually the natural habit of sleep. Anthropologic scientists have established that the way we sleep in modern civilization is artificial. Our ancestors' sleep pattern or "Paleo Sleep" consisted of sleeping in two parts. The early part was when the "work of the day" was done, a light cold meal, followed by a sleep for a few hours before getting up for a larger hot meal. After this larger meal they would go back to sleep until daylight woke them up.

Ultimately, I'll do whatever it takes to be the doctor I was born to be. My desire to provide the very best care to my patients is insatiable. My love for them is limitless.

Intense? You bet it's intense! But, you must understand, this isn't just a job for me. It's far more than a "forty hours a week" or "9:00-5:00 each day" career. Medicine is many things for different people. Of course it's a profession for some, a calling or career for others, maybe even a hobby for a few. But to me, it is my life! It's the guiding purpose I sense in every cell of my body and I'm very serious about it.

This intensity, this passion has caused me a good bit of difficulty through the years in connecting with my associates in the medical field. Their dreams often revolve around getting their practices to the point where they can actually work less and see fewer patients. Some long for quitting time to roll around so they can leave the office and get to the driving range to work on their golf swing. Others put in the eighty to one hundred hours a week so they can take a week off every month and enjoy the fruits of their labor. Many take a mid-week day off. They spend weekends at their cabins at the lake…a just reward for their week's effort. For them, medicine is simply a vehicle to reach other goals; their real passions and desires lay elsewhere.

BORN TO BE A DOCTOR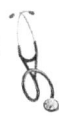

Of course much of this is not their fault. They've been shaped by the way formal medicine has progressed, or in my view, regressed. Gone are the days of the horse and buggy doctor who treated his or her patients with care and gut instinct based on lots of study and real life examples. Most of today's doctors have merely become health care providers. They're forced to serve the big pharmaceutical and insurance companies leaving little room in their practices for actually serving the patient. Their reliance on new technologies has put them out of touch with what the patient really needs, a doctor who cares. Sadly, all this results in a less productive practice, and in many cases, a less enjoyable life for the physician.

I apologize if I'm overly critical, but this type of medical practice doesn't fit my experience at all. For years, I've had some colleagues pontificate about their practice, telling me I could have much more time to enjoy my family and make more money if I only did things their way.

But unlike so many in medicine today, money is not a motivator for me. My only desire is to pay my expenses and continue to have a venue to see and help patients. My early trauma and difficulty in school taught me to break everything down to a simplified set of instructions so that I could easily understand. In many ways, being a poor student made me a good teacher. So much so that I was awarded Teacher of the Year in my first year of teaching at a UCLA medical school!

IT'S ABOUT THE CARE OF THE PATIENT

The way my practice is organized, I see fewer patients by design, and, for this reason, make less money. But seeing fewer

The Good Doctor

patients allows me more time with each patient. At least that's the way it's supposed to work. It's hard for me to limit the number of folks I see. I'm always ready to see one more patient or spend just a few more minutes listening to their stories. Consequently, it's not odd for me to be at the office until after 8:00 p.m. This extra time not only helps me make a better diagnosis, it helps me build relationships and bond with my patients, which is important to me.

Until recently, after office hours, I would go to the hospital until 11:00 p.m., eating a quick bite on the way home. I'd arrive home to a dark house with everyone sound asleep. I'd go straight to bed for an hour or two before getting up for the most important few hours of my day, reading and studying to keep pace with the current research. Then, like I talked about, I would go back to sleep for a couple of hours. Overnight phone calls and trips back to the hospital for emergencies would interrupt my study and sleep at times, but I never minded it much. I was doing what I loved and I was thriving! In my first real practice in Sedalia, Missouri, I once went sixteen months without a single day off. I was the only board certified internist for a region with a population of over 100,000 souls. In those days I was more a cardiologist than any other area of special training on my "dance card." It was while at that post in Sedalia that I put in the first pacemaker, started the first Cardiac Intensive Care Unit and ICU for our regional hospital. It's no wonder I felt responsible to personally be there to supervise all that was going on at the time.

Many doctors operate clinics that are more like medical mills chewing up four to five patients an hour in order to pay for their massive overhead. Quick solutions or shuffling patients off for one more test or procedure seems to be the

BORN TO BE A DOCTOR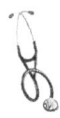

order of the day. Think about it, when was the last time you heard someone crow about how much they loved their doctor and treasured the time they spent with him or her?

It's time to face the fact that something is broken in the way most doctors practice medicine.

Looking back, my practice has been an unrelenting search for answers for the patients in my care. I believe that God has put this fire down deep in my being. He created me to do this. He's the one who has blessed me so that I can fulfill my passion and it's Him I'm accountable to. Believe me, I feel the weight of that truth every single day. That's why it's hard for me to take time off or spend my time doing anything else but seeing to the needs of my patients. Because of this passion, I'm driven, single-minded, and laser focused.

Being a doctor has meant spending a lifetime in the midst of the human experience. I've been there for the soaring highs and the tragic and terrible lows. Like the horse and buggy doctors who came before me, I've been deeply involved in the lives of my patients—many of whom have become close friends through the years.

I've had to watch patients die regardless of what I did to stave off death. I've felt the helplessness of finding no answers and having to admit to family members that I had no idea why their loved one died while someone else in similar straits lived. I detest death and disease and have committed my life to defeating these enemies at every turn, realizing that the biggest adversary is not the patient's genetics but rather their lifestyle superimposed on their age that causes most of the problems.

That's why it's so heartbreaking to admit the times I didn't possess the proper weapons to win the battle on their behalf. I

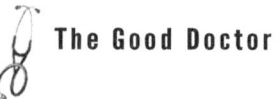

The Good Doctor

could never just shrug my shoulders and say to myself, "Death happens every day. It's part of the circle of life." You see, to me it's huge. I always feel the defeat deeply whenever I've lost a battle for one of my patients. The loss drives me back to the books to study and learn new solutions, develop new weapons and strategies so we can be more successful next time.

I strive to arm the people I treat with the knowledge and motivation to alter their way of life. I provide articles and books I have written, radio and television programs I have done, as well as the many lectures I have given over the years. Unfortunately, these efforts have largely fallen on deaf ears. People have always had a hard time accepting the role they play in their own health care. I have spent a lifetime stressing to all my patients that they are the ones most responsible for their health. The things they eat, their exercise (or lack of it), their stress levels, even their outlook, whether positive or negative, all contribute mightily to their health, even more than their own genetics.

But I've been blessed to see the other side as well. I saw the light that beams from faces when they are told that the tests are negative or that the disease that threatened so mightily has been defeated. Fortunately, often I've been able to give the right answer at just the right time to bridge the gap between disease and healing. I've watched patients who had been given only months to live by a specialist, go on to live many more productive years because of a new strategy for their disease that we embarked upon together. Thank God!

That is why I'm a doctor.

That's why I spend countless hours every week, even to this day, studying in order to learn new ways to bring solace and

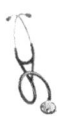

healing to my patients—not just the traditional, tried and true methods but alternative and even experimental methods. Whatever it takes to defeat the enemies or devils that ravage my patients and friends. That's why I've sacrificed so much through the years. That's what keeps the fire in my belly burning brightly, even now after fifty-plus years of practicing medicine.

Continuing medical education is now and was a mandate for me even before graduating from medical school. Most of the "medicine" was traditional but I wanted more. Arcane, different for sure, but obtaining this information back then was much more difficult since the material was not taught in formal medical institutions. Add to that the fact that the purveyors were at odds with the "straights" who formally taught at the medical schools and the national recognized colleges of specialties such as mine, The American College of Medicine, or for my surgical colleagues, The American College of Surgeons. These were the carefully groomed children of the grand American Board of Medical Specialties. They fostered the traditional educators from well-known medical schools. But what they taught was usually just a rehash of what I had read in the medical journals. I wanted more.

To gain this "inside information" I would seek out a physician who published such medical articles in non-peer reviewed journals or even in self-published books that at times would be a best seller like Dr. Robert Atkins.

Rarely, and if living close to my practice, I would take him to dinner and "pick" lots from his brain and only a little of the food. Even a better ploy, which I did many times in the 70s, was to seek out a notable physician and offer to pay him an honorarium of $500-$1000 a day to let me shadow him in his medical practice. Of course I paid my flights, room and board

The Good Doctor

as well as hire a doctor to watch my practice while I was in my new training program.

Soon after I started private practice, I became interested in chelation medicine. I read articles, books and then was introduced to the American Board of Chelation Therapy (now the ABCMT), which required a weekend course and a score of 65 percent on a five-hour written examination. It was through this group that I met their leadership sponsor, ACAM (American College of the Advancement of Medicine). I went to several of their national meetings, but was not impressed by the lectures in that they were more junk science rather than the academic methodology that was more my style. Then I heard of Capitol University of Integrated Medicine in Washington, DC.

Capital University of Integrative Medicine (CUIM) was founded in 1995 to provide education for medical and health practitioners wishing to incorporate integrative therapies from multiple disciplines of medicine within their practices. Responding to the demands of both practitioners and patients, CUIM embraced a simple but progressive mission to encourage health care professionals to promote health assessment and advance integrative therapies to improve quality of life, alleviate illness, prevent chronic degenerative diseases, and reduce premature death.

The University founders held that Americans desire and deserve the opportunity to receive the highest quality of health care with the broadest range of safe and effective care options. In keeping with this belief, CUIM's mission was to educate and develop health care professionals, including those currently practicing, to serve the public. The University dedicated itself to bringing insight and offering encouragement to those

BORN TO BE A DOCTOR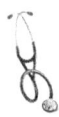

interested in exploring various forms of health assessment and patient-centered therapeutics.

From 1996 to 2006, CUIM served as a licensed graduate professional university and the only resident institution of higher education in the United States with a curriculum of widely diverse integrative health therapies. Following a decade of service, CUIM graduated its final class of students and closed in June 2006.

From its inception, the University consistently promoted advancement of integrative health and healing through education and research. The noble aims of Capital University of Integrative Medicine still continue through its many graduates and faculty.

Their philosophy, like mine, places the patient at the center of the health care team. The degree was a thorough, three full days a month, twenty-four month program for already medically credentialed candidates. The professors were the same doctors that I sought in my private curriculum of the decades of traveling throughout the world to achieve my personal goal of learning to become a "good doctor."

In the previous years I did spend a fair amount of time both teaching and learning at several formal German medical institutions. At graduation, not only did we have to successfully pass the required classes and written tests, but to write, defend, and publish a thesis on an academic research project. This was my "cup of tea"! I could meet, learn, and socialize with professionals who were like-minded. No longer did I have to travel to the various cities to study, but could do so in a central location, Washington, DC, on a monthly basis. Both their colleagues and students would get together to learn and teach.

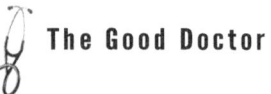# The Good Doctor

In 1997, I enrolled and, along with twelve other doctors, continued my integrated medical education. There were courses such as Homeopathy, Oriental Medicine, Vibratory Medicine, Herbal Medicine, Nutritional Medicine as well as mainstream with an integrative approach were to be learned.

Indeed, I learned from these innovative professors as well as my fellow students the fine art and science of this amalgam of the "new medicine." Fortunately, I was president of my class, and wrote and defended my thesis ("The Autonomic Effects for an aromatic essential oil, Sandalwood on Health") gathering as much other medical information as I could to better the health of my current and future patients. I not only graduated but also stayed on for two more years as a professor to teach the incoming students what I had learned and perfected in this type of medicine.

I did have a choice in my degree to be awarded a Doctor of Integrated Medicine, DIM, or a Master's degree in Medicine that I was told was like a PhD. Since I did not want to be DIM, I chose the latter. It is this document that now hangs on my wall of academic degrees along with my collection of Bachelor's, Medical Doctor, and the various specialty degrees that have been awarded to me.

Being a doctor is not just what I do. It's who I am. I think, breathe, and live it each and every day, even on days when I'm not in the office. There is no backing away, slowing down, or retiring from this kind of calling. Sound religious? It is! I believe that, in many ways, medicine is just as much religion as it is science. Both require a great deal of faith.

I'm called to be a doctor...until the day I die, and maybe afterward!

CHAPTER THREE:

A FATHER'S INFLUENCE

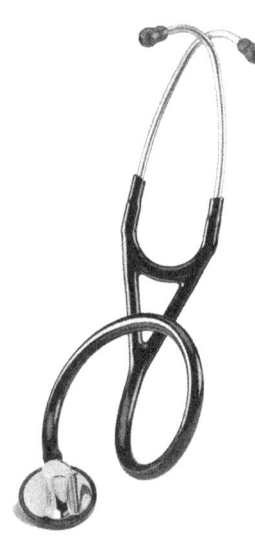

I was born to be a doctor.

But it didn't happen overnight. It took a tremendous amount of hard work. It was my destiny, but I still had to endure a lot of sleepless nights and stressful days. I guess it's just my nature that the things I want so desperately in life have not always come easily. There has been a lot of sacrifice over the years. My devotion to medicine has been all consuming, probably to a fault.

How did it all begin? How did the events and circumstances of my life conspire to make me into the doctor, into the man I am today? I may have been born to be a doctor, but I didn't just step from childhood into the medical practice. Now, with the perspective of age and hindsight, I can see God's hand has directed me, guided me along this path. His hand has been on my shoulder all along life's journey.

We're all influenced to some degree by the environment in which we've grown up. Our family, our friends, our teachers,

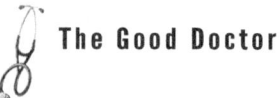
The Good Doctor

our hometown and neighborhood all leave their indelible mark on our lives in one way or another.

As I look back over my life and the choices and decisions I made, I can see the undeniable influence of Charlie Block, my father. He loomed as a larger-than-life figure in my life.

As a young boy, I noticed that there were two things in life that really piqued my father's interest, making money to support his family and medicine. I saw him achieve a few great things in his life, all because of his commitment to hard work. There was nothing he was unwilling to do to provide for his family. I'm convinced that my own work ethic and my deep desire to become a doctor came directly from my father.

WORKING ON THE RAILROAD

I was born in Philadelphia but I was raised, from the time I was three years old, in Atlantic City, New Jersey. My dad was originally from Philadelphia and my mom was from Atlantic City. The two cities are only about sixty miles apart and connected by a train named the "Atlantic City Line," which is now part of the New Jersey Transit Authority. The train ride from one city to the other takes about an hour and forty-five minutes and when it was time for us to move, we simply went from one end of the line to the other.

The train was an important part of our lives. The Atlantic City Line is where my father went to work every day. He didn't have much of an education (he did not graduate from the sixth grade), but what he didn't get from a formal education, he made up for with tireless ambition and hard work. He started working on the trains before WWII, selling orange juice and

A FATHER'S INFLUENCE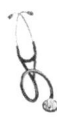

bologna sandwiches to commuters riding the train. But when the war started late in 1941, everything changed.

The trains were now carrying many more passengers, and not just commuters. The trains brought new recruits to the Navy bases located further to the south in Maryland. My dad's bosses offered him a position on the train running from Perryville, Maryland, to the important ports and military bases at Bay Bridge.

The train stations along the route would overflow with 12,000 to 15,000 new recruits arriving every day or so. They moved my father off the train and let him put a little stand in the train station at Perryville. In those days with the war on, there were severe shortages on even the most ordinary things. Sometimes the things people wanted most were difficult to come by—like chewing gum, butter, cheese, and rubber products. It was from the latter that my father's income greatly benefited. He sold chewing gum and condoms that were both hard to come by in those days. He would hawk to the Naval recruits, "Chew and Screw them for a Two 'em!" It may not sound like much by today's standards, but my father was able to make between $35,000 and $40,000 a year selling the most common things out of that little stand.

One of the things that impacted me most was his desire to bring me along to help him. I would do anything to be alongside my dad and I loved working with him. I'd help him make sandwiches and the orange slush drinks that we'd sell out of the little stand. Working alongside him allowed me to observe and learn the ways in which he made his money.

It wasn't long before I yearned to go into business for myself. I saw what making money meant to my father. I saw the

The Good Doctor

independence it brought him and his family. That's what I wanted. I never really wanted to live better or to be rich. Money wasn't a motivator to me. It was just a tool, a tool that would ultimately enable me to attend college and later medical school. I was miserly on spending anything on myself. I was focused on saving all I could in order to have my heart's desire, to be a doctor.

JOINING THE WORKFORCE

When I was only about seven years old, I got my first official job selling newspapers. At the time, the mid 1940s, Atlantic City was in its heyday and was known as America's Great Convention City. The streets were packed with tourists in the summer and the locals, in lesser numbers, in the off-season.

My strategy was to go to one of the main streets, which was full of bars and taverns and saloons. I'd sell newspapers to the folks hanging out there. I worked every night from 6:30 until about 9:00.

I would buy the paper for a nickel and sell them for seven cents. To make it easy, most of the customers would just give me a dime, some even a quarter. They thought it was cute to have such a young kid selling papers and, of course, I made the most of it!

I don't think there are too many parents today who would let their seven year old go from bar to bar selling newspapers to strangers each evening after dinner. But that was a different day and age, and my folks knew I was doing more than just earning money. I was busy learning the value of hard work and saving for the future instead of spending it on short-term,

A FATHER'S INFLUENCE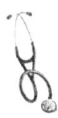

selfish gratification. I knew I wanted to be a doctor and that motivated me to save as much as I could for college.

When I turned eleven years old, I switched from selling newspapers at night to selling ice cream and popsicles during the day until it got dark. I was hired to ride a little cart that I would pedal up and down the street, ringing my bell to alert the kids I was coming. But soon I found a way to make even more money.

There was an older boy selling what we called "snowballs." A snowball was a cup filled with chopped ice with syrup of various flavors poured over the top. This kid was actually sponsored by a pharmacy whose owner wanted to make a little extra money. One day, when the boy got sick, I asked to take his place until he got better. He never did come back, and I worked the rest of the summer selling snowballs. The profit margin was much higher for snowballs instead of ice cream. My take doubled from 20 percent to 40 percent.

It was easy to keep the accounting straight when you were selling ice cream because they were single-serving bowls that came in boxes of twelve. But the chopped ice for snowballs was sold to the pharmacy in fifty-pound bags. The way we kept track of sales was by counting the cups. At the end of the day, I'd reconcile the number of cups I took out by the number of cups I brought back and that way I'd know what the sales number was. I would split the profits with the pharmacy owner accordingly. His share was six cents per cup. The snowballs were sold in cone-shaped cups that came in a sleeve with fifty cups in each sleeve.

Because it was common to have a few cups blow away or get lost during the day, he allowed me five "free cups" every day. But one day disaster struck when the cups in one sleeve became twisted, ruining the whole sleeve except the top four or five cups. Under the top five cups, which appeared to be just fine, the whole rest of the sleeve was twisted, ruining the rest of the cups in the sleeve, making them unusable.

I explained what happened, but the pharmacist didn't believe me! I threw the mess out and paid the pharmacist for just the five cups I used. He blew his stack and accused me of cheating him! He said I'd stolen from him and demanded I pay him for the full sleeve of cups. Grudgingly, I paid the man even though my take for the whole day was less than a couple of bucks. For me, it wasn't even about the money. What bothered me most was being accused of cheating him out of money. I knew it was time to make a change!

It was about this time I began thinking about starting my own business. Since selling snowballs was much more profitable than selling ice cream, I knew that's the direction I wanted to go. With my father's help, I bought an ice cream cart bicycle chassis and converted it with the help of a sheet metal worker to become my new Snowball cart.

Over the years, I added an OrangeAide server and was able to sell hotdogs. It didn't take long until my cart weighed 500 pounds. As soon as I was old enough to drive, I motorized the whole contraption. I used this vending cart every summer until I was a sophomore in medical school. By the time my junior year in high school rolled around I had purchased a luncheonette in a bowling alley. This became my "winter business." I ran the luncheonette business after school every night until the leagues were finished. I worked weekends too.

As I look back, it seems like an incredible amount of maturity and business acumen for a kid of eleven years old to have.

A FATHER'S INFLUENCE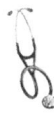

But that's all due to my father's influence. I became industrious because of the example he set. He taught me that if I wanted to get ahead in life, I had to do more than just dream about it. I would have to work very hard. His example taught me that I was going to need to set a goal and not let anything get in the way of achieving that objective. I began to enjoy what having money would mean in my life. I was popular and respected by my friends because I could make so much money.

But my business went to the next level when I brought in my friends to work for me. I increased my sales force with three other boys. We put all the ice and the bottles of flavoring in boxes that the guys could carry on their shoulders. Then I would take my team out on the beach to sell to the crowds there. I would give them half of everything they made. This was a real eye-opening transition for me. I was learning to not just be industrious; I was learning to be entrepreneurial. I began to see that if I hired guys to work for me I could multiply myself and increase my profits!

MY FATHER'S MEDICAL STRUGGLE

If it was my father's hard work ethic that provided my motivation, it was his intense interest in medicine that gave me direction. From the time I was very young, he was obsessed with learning more about the various ailments, either real or imagined from which he suffered. Although he was keenly interested in medicine, he knew there was no way for him to become a doctor himself...he had dropped out of school before making it to junior high.

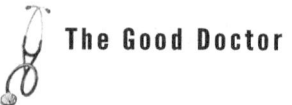
The Good Doctor

My father's medical curiosity was born out of the fact that he was a hypochondriac; he believed he was afflicted with a host of ailments. I can't count the number of times he would talk to me about all of his medical problems. All the things that were wrong with him mystified him. His desire to learn more and more about medicine was limitless. He would pour over magazines and newspaper articles written by doctors. He believed doctors were God-like; having super-human knowledge of all there was to know about the physical condition. It was this admiration of physicians that caused me to look up to and respect them as well.

When I was only eight years old, my father told me that he had an incurable disease called Paget's disease. Fear gripped me. I was seized with the terror of losing my dad. I was convinced that my hero could die any day! As a little boy, I had yet to learn the difference between the words "incurable" and "fatal."

My dad did, in fact, suffer from Paget's disease, which is a chronic disorder that can result in enlarged and misshapen bones. Caused by the breakdown of the bones, Paget's is often followed by disorganized and uneven bone re-formation. The end result is that the affected bone is weakened, resulting in severe pain, misshapen bones, fractures, and arthritis in the joints near the bones affected by the disease.

In my father's case, he was diagnosed in 1942 after slipping on the ice on his way to work at the train station. His leg was badly broken. That marked the beginning of his lifelong battle with Paget's disease. Over his lifetime, he suffered over twenty-six fractures. Each painful fracture served to make his bones thicker and smaller, causing him to lose six inches in

A FATHER'S INFLUENCE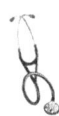

height and become hunched over and unable to look us in the face. By the time he died at eighty-two, he was only 4'9".

His interest in the medical profession and his curiosity about what was going on in his own body never wavered. The seeds of that curiosity were instilled in me early on; my father taught me that doctors were highly respected and had answers that could help others. I grew up believing that doctors were imbued with a special kind of wisdom. They had ways of unlocking the mysteries of health, disease, death, and the human body. I was very young, but I knew my destiny beyond a shadow of a doubt. I was born to be a doctor.

My father wasn't the lone influencer in my life. As a young boy, I would get sick often and Dr. Leonard Erber, our family doctor, would come to our house and give me a shot. I didn't know what was in the injection, but I knew that Dr. Erber had the power to make me feel better. This, combined with my father's high opinion of doctors, confirmed to me that's what I wanted to do when I grew up. I wanted to help people. I wanted to help them feel better.

Dr. Erber was an enormous influence in my life. He had a medical practice, but he also worked at one of the hospitals in Atlantic City. I finally worked up the courage to ask him what I needed to do in order to become a physician. He told me there were two things I had to do: work hard and do well in school. The working hard part would be easy. I knew I could do that. It was doing well in school that was going to be a challenge.

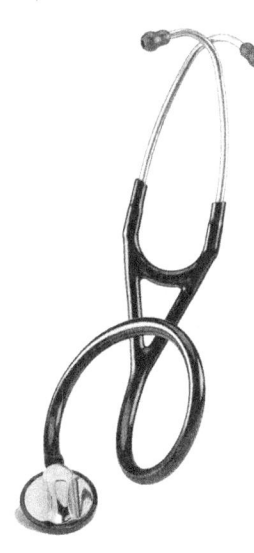

CHAPTER FOUR:

THE SCHOOL YEARS

I learned the power of a strong commitment early in life. I've always admired marathon runners. At that extreme distance, the runners must be able to endure a tremendous amount of hardship during the race in order to finish. Most anyone who can run at all can run a 100-meter dash, but it's not as easy to run 26.2 miles, even for the elite athletes. The successful ones aren't just the ones in the best physical shape; they're the ones who are strong mentally and able to overcome adversity.

Of course, life is often compared to the marathon. Those who are able to succeed in life and finish well are the ones who are able to push through even when things are tough. The ones who are willing to do whatever it takes are the ones who get ahead...and stay ahead.

With the influence of my father and Dr. Erber, I believed I was ready to do whatever it took to become a doctor. Like the marathon runner, I was prepared to endure through to the finish. When my parents found out about my goal they were very pleased but told me right up front that there was no way they were going to be able to afford to send me to college, let alone medical school. I knew then that if I was going to accomplish this lofty goal, I was going to have to pay my own way.

I told everyone I encountered I wanted to become a doctor. I had some serious challenges. I could work hard but I was such a poor student, I knew I was going to have a difficult time with the schooling. Most folks who heard about my goal assumed it was just a pie in the sky dream, one that didn't stand a chance of coming true.

SHAPED FROM BIRTH

My parents came by their skepticism honestly, both having come from very difficult backgrounds. I was their first child and couldn't help but be on the receiving end of their inexperience and immaturity. From the time I was born, I was caught in a perfect storm of dysfunction and disorder.

Simply put, neither of my parents was prepared to have a child. As a child, my mother was spoiled, doted on by a father and grandparents after her own mother died when my mother was only nine years old. My dad grew up with a profound sense of self-sufficiency thrust on him after his own father abandoned him, ironically, when he was nine years old. He was forced to live with foster parents until he finally ran away from home, living and providing for himself even from a young age.

The early years of their own marriage was filled with turmoil. That is the world in which I was conceived. My mind was programmed by this dysfunction during development while I was still in the womb. Even in utero I couldn't escape

THE SCHOOL YEARS

the feelings of strife and disappointment. My mother's family was never convinced that my father was good enough for her. The pressure they put on my parents created unbearable stress. Instead of a blessing, their new pregnancy became a curse, an undesirable detour in their young lives. As a result, there is no doubt I was unwanted from the start. My parents argued non-stop. I was exposed to this contention and strife as a fetus and it shaped the way I felt about myself from birth.

It's no wonder I was born feeling that I was a bad baby, a terrible toddler, and a monster child. To add to the devastating emotional abandonment by my mother, my father blamed me for my mom's depressed emotional state. Today, my mother's condition would easily be diagnosed as postpartum depression brought on by a progesterone deficiency. But in those days, no one knew about those concepts, which today have helped so many of my own patients, not to mention the tens of thousands of other doctors' patients.

But in my home, I became a lightning rod, a point of focus for both my parents' anger. As a child, I knew that in order to survive in that contentious environment, I was going to have to become a fighter myself. I think that's why, even as an adult, I tend to kick against the establishment.

This tendency created a lot of problems during my growing up years at home. I drove my parents, and, in particular, my father who was an overreactor with limited education, to such emotional upset and distraction. They knew they were going to have to do something with me to save what was left of their sanity.

Because they truly felt they were already doing all they could, they decided to get me out of the house instead of digging deeper and giving me the love I so desperately craved. Because of that decision, I struggle to this day with feelings that I don't have enough love to keep my soul satisfied.

In their immaturity and pain, they decided their only option was to put me in the care of a foster family. I was placed with a "professional" foster family who made their living keeping kids for the state. Ironically, their name was Foster.

It's terribly tragic to me even now in the retelling. My mother and father didn't even tell me that I was going to go live with another family. They simply got up one morning and said that they were going on a vacation with my younger brother and since I couldn't miss any school, I was going to have to stay with the Fosters. I had no idea what the truth really was until early one day on the way to school, in a moment of overwhelming homesickness I decided to make a short detour. I would make a quick stop over at my old house instead of going straight to school. I told myself I would only stay a moment. I just wanted to be surrounded by familiarity for a bit in a place I knew well.

I went to the house expecting it to be empty. But it wasn't. My parents and my younger brother were there, all playing together in my parents' bed. It was like a punch to the gut. I was stunned and ran out of the house still trying to process the lie and betrayal of my parents. My grief and confusion had reached an all-new low. No matter what I tried, there was no way I could get my family to love me.

TROUBLE AT SCHOOL

Unfortunately, my problems at home followed me to school. I was a difficult and defiant student. I guess in that way, the

THE SCHOOL YEARS

money I made as a boy had a negative effect. I thought I was above school. I had proven I didn't need the education to make good money. But I still clung to the dream of becoming a doctor, and I knew in order for that dream to come true, I was going to have to be a good student.

My problems with school started early on. My birthday is in February, so I was six months younger than most other students in my class. For that reason, I was always one of the smaller kids in my grade. I was overweight and got called a lot of names, including "Fatty." I was picked on and bullied endlessly. Even at that age, I resolved never to grow up to be obese...and so far so good!

To add to my problems, I had Attention Deficit Disorder or ADD and my teachers didn't think I even had the capacity to learn. At the time, there was no designation of ADD; kids like me were just called underachievers or just plain dumb. There simply wasn't the awareness of these conditions among teachers then like there is today. I was continually left behind in favor of the kids who were able to learn more quickly and adapt to the classroom setting more easily. I struggled so much, in fact, that my parents held me back in the fifth grade.

Being held back ended up being a blessing in disguise. I went from being one of the smallest and dumbest kids in my class to being one of the better students (at least for a year). As a result, I started to build relationships with a whole set of new friends. I went from being outcast to being looked up to as one of the leaders of my gang of new friends. Because of my lingering insecurities, I thought I had to have a gimmick. In those days, we wrote everything in ink, using fountain pens. To keep the ink close by, everyone had an inkwell in his or her desk. I

The Good Doctor

never had good hand-eye coordination and would spill my ink all over the desk and myself when I wrote. Others would see my mess and accuse me of drinking the ink since it would invariably end up all over my face. Of course, I never did taste the ink, let alone drink it, but it was something no one else did. So I embraced and embellished it and took on the persona of someone different and unique. It paid off. I became a popular kid. The kids in my class were fascinated with me and thought it would be cool to be friends with such an eccentric.

CHUCKY AND ME

Of course, I'll have to admit, this wasn't always a positive thing. Looking back, I can see that I wasn't always a good influence on the other kids. Chucky Kahn is a prime example.

Chucky and I were actually born on the same day, but our paths didn't cross again until we were in the same prekindergarten class. I still remember our teacher was Mrs. McClosky. We were only four years old but we became fast friends. As we grew older, our paths diverged. He grew up in a wealthier part of Atlantic City, while our home was in a poorer section of Absecon Island, in which Atlantic City occupied most of the real estate.

As I mentioned, I grew up in the rough and tumble streets of Atlantic City. I would spend my evenings selling newspapers in the bars on the streets of the city. I knew my way around and developed a keen sense of just how much trouble I could get into without getting caught.

My upbringing was a lot different than Chucky's much more sheltered childhood. Chucky's home life was much more

THE SCHOOL YEARS

stable than mine. When with me, Chucky undoubtedly saw another side of life. To this day, Chucky blames me for introducing him to a whole new level of mischief. We had a lot of fun, even though much of it was against the law! Over the years, I was the one who introduced Chucky to gambling, girls, drag racing, and underage drinking. Chucky and I were inseparable. I brought him the excitement and thrill that his life lacked, and he brought me the stability, balance, consistency, and confidence that I didn't get at home. When I was around Chucky, I felt that if I tried hard and didn't give up I could do whatever I put my mind to.

In fact, it was Chucky's father who became another primary influence in my life. Dr. Leo Kahn was a pillar in the community. My dad had always looked up to doctors and looking through his eyes, I could easily see how respected Dr. Kahn was around town. This made an enormous impact on me in my early years. I would often spend weekends with Chucky and his family. Dr. Kahn, who was a general practitioner, would talk to me long into the night about his practice. He would speak in detail about his commitment to medicine. I could sense his deep passion for his patients. It was easy to get swept up in his zeal. My dad's respect for doctors, coupled with real live examples like Dr. Erber and Dr. Kahn, helped cement in my mind the desire to be a doctor.

But for the longest time, it looked like my goal might be just talk. Holding me back a grade in school helped me make friends and fit in more comfortably, but it did nothing for me academically. Even though I was trying my hardest, I still had failing grades.

The Good Doctor

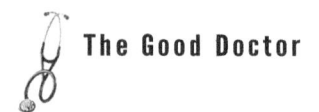

GETTING ON TRACK

However, by the time I got to high school, in algebra class, something finally clicked. I don't know what happened, but after failing class after class I actually got a B! After that, I took geometry and got the highest mark of all the classes in my grade! Of course, the teachers were immediately skeptical. They summoned me to the principal's office and accused me of cheating, but I knew better. That kind of math had just clicked, and I knew from that day forward I'd be okay, at least in mathematical concepts.

But my success in math didn't extend to the other subjects. I was barely able to pass my other classes. My grades were horrible, and I felt like a failure. Not surprisingly, I was in the bottom 20 percent of the class. With my miserable grades and low class ranking, I knew my chances of getting into college were slim, to say the least. I wanted to be a doctor more than anything else so I went to see the career counselors at school to see if there was some way they could help me. Surprisingly, all they did was to try to talk me out of becoming a doctor, instead of encouraging me to do something more obtainable, like becoming a teacher. Ironically, the word "doctor" in Latin is *dicere*, which means "to teach or say."

They gave me a placement exam to help determine what kind of aptitude I had for different types of careers. They'd asked questions like, "If you had a typewriter, would you rather type on it, or sell it, or fix it?" After hearing the options, I figured I would prefer to either sell the typewriter or repair it. I knew I didn't want to type on it! So after seeing the results of the test, they said I should probably try to be a teacher or

THE SCHOOL YEARS

social worker. They continued to discourage me from the physician's path.

When it was time to take the college entrance exams, I bought a study guide to help me prepare for the test. Chucky was a tremendous help to me. Studying came much more easily for him, and he encouraged me to prepare for the college boards. For four weeks I got up much earlier than usual and spent at least two hours studying before class just to prepare for that test.

The study handbook for the test was divided up into the two sections that would ultimately make up the formal test. I chose to not even look at the math section, realizing that with mathematics, either a person is born with that God-given aptitude or not. Based on my high school success, I figured I had that gift whether my teachers believed the notion or not. There was a ten thousand word dictionary in the College Board Test Guide. I buckled down to accomplish that feat.

By the time I took the test I practically had that whole dictionary memorized. Again, hard work never intimidated me. If memorizing an entire book was what I had to do to get into college, then that's what I was going to do. It was a "have to or die" situation and being distracted was not an option. With Chucky's help, I was learning how to focus for the first time in my academic career.

I took the test and scored in the top 2 percentile of students in reading and comprehension. In math, I was in the top 1 percentile! I guess I remembered most of the words in the study guide dictionary (and still do sixty years later!). Fortunately, the math section wasn't actually arithmetic at all, but rather

The Good Doctor

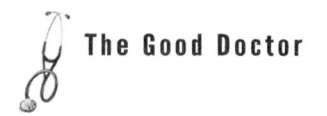

a series of complicated number games that I was able to do well on.

OFF TO COLLEGE

But, unfortunately, a high grade on the entrance exam did not guarantee a spot in a great school. In those years following WWII, it was tough to get into college. The GI's returning home were able to go to college on the GI Bill and flooded freshmen classes at colleges across the country. Enrollment at colleges and universities swelled and made few available spots for guys like me. In those days, they didn't have "feeder schools" like junior colleges or community colleges to help students like me get to the next academic level.

Many of the schools I was most interested in wouldn't even take a second look at me. But there was one school willing to take a chance. The school was Muhlenberg College in Allentown, Pennsylvania, about 130 miles from my home in Atlantic City. I knew it was going to be tough, but their belief in me made my confidence soar. I was ready to give my all to prove to them that choosing me wasn't a mistake.

Muhlenberg had one of the premier pre-med programs in the country. In fact, at the time, they boasted a 100 percent acceptance rate into medical school. What I didn't know is that if I were unable to maintain an excellent GPA, I would be summarily removed from the pre-med program and not receive their recommendation for medical school. All I knew and all I cared about at the time was that I had cleared the first major hurdle in my quest to become a doctor. I was the first in my family in a generation to go to college.

THE SCHOOL YEARS

I was thrilled to get to Muhlenberg. To make my transition just that much easier, I was able to room with my old friend, Chucky Kahn. He, like his father, went to the University of Pennsylvania a year earlier (he wasn't held back in school like I was) and switched to Muhlenberg to be with me.

The very first test that first semester was in History of Civilization. I flunked the test only scoring a meager 36 percent! I knew college was going to be a big challenge for me, but I had no idea it was going to be this hard. There was no way I was going to be able to stay in school with grades like that. The first month in college wasn't even over, and my dream of becoming a doctor was already in grave jeopardy.

That first test reduced me to tears. What a disaster! How was I ever going to become a doctor? I couldn't even pass a simple history test! Once again, I turned to Chucky for help. I told him I was reading all the reading assignments, familiarizing myself with all my lecture notes before every test, and still not doing well.

Right off, he told me to forget about only reading and familiarizing myself with the material. He reminded me of the success I had on the college entrance exam. If I wanted to succeed in college, I was going to have to do the very same thing I did for that test. I was going to have to knuckle down and memorize all the material!

I immediately switched my study strategies. Now I would spend every hour I could memorizing the material for every class. Chucky and I lived in an apartment together, and that's where I would spend almost all my waking hours when not at school or at work studying.

The Good Doctor

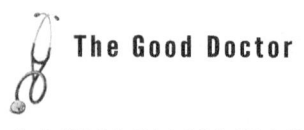

A NEW CHALLENGE

I knew how to work hard to get what I wanted. But now I was going to have to work extra hard. I'd met a girl and this was before birth control pills, so we had to get married. So now, instead of just needing to earn enough money to support myself, I had someone else to support as well. But that wasn't my only challenge with the upcoming marriage. I was Jewish, and while not orthodox, the faith was very important to my parents. My new fianceé was not Jewish, and I knew this had the potential of causing big problems for my mom and dad. I encouraged her to convert to Judaism. We eloped, lied about our ages and got married by a justice of the peace. Our marriage had a rough start but soon enough my family came to accept her especially after her conversion. It did take a little longer for her family to accept me and their daughter's conversion to Judaism.

Our family soon expanded with our first child, a daughter, Vici. As much as I loved my family, the new responsibilities were beginning to weigh heavily on my shoulders. Our new baby represented a new mouth to feed. I loved and cared deeply for my family, but I also needed to finish college before attending medical school. I was being tugged in many conflicting directions; family, maintaining good grades in pre-med school, and earning a living were all constantly vying for my time and attention. It's easy now, in hindsight, to see the instances when I sacrificed valuable time with my family in favor of my passion for my career. I'm sorry now to say that my young family didn't get nearly the attention from me that they needed. I have regrets to this day, but despite that adversity, my family did thrive, once again proving that nurture is stronger than nature.

THE SCHOOL YEARS

POUNDING THE PAVEMENT

By the time I became a senior in college, I had found myself carrying a very full and challenging pre-med course load while still needing to work close to full-time hours just to support my family. In order to make the money we needed to survive, I worked almost full time selling things. Just like when I was a kid, I sold snowballs early in the day and sold books and encyclopedias door-to-door in the evening. I was fortunate enough to be successful, so much so that the book company gave me my own team of salesmen. My new team strategy was to take five young students and drop them off on a city block. I would circle back around and pick them up a few hours later.

This strategy worked well. Early on, the company started sending me to small towns as part of a team to sell the encyclopedias. This was in an area of Pennsylvania known widely for its coal production. There was a tremendous amount of coal mined in the hills around my college. This was in the Lehigh Valley with the two principal cities of Allentown, where Muhlenberg was located, and Bethlehem, which was known for its steel production. The coal mined out of those mountains was used to make the steel. It takes almost a ton of coal to make a ton of steel.

Coal mining was hard work, and the work bred hard people, not easy to sell to door-to-door. To make matters worse, they weren't selling much coal in those days and prices were dropping. Mines were going out of business and people were losing their jobs. These small towns were losing their populations to the bigger cities. It was a bleak time in the hills of Pennsylvania.

The Good Doctor

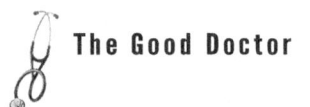

I learned firsthand just how tough it could be trying to sell encyclopedias to folks who barely had the money to buy food and were faced with the very real possibility of losing their homes. They were hardly willing to spend what precious little they had on something as seemingly frivolous as a set of new encyclopedias.

The hardship made me rethink and come up with a new sales strategy. I came up with a whole new sales pitch for my team. When I would approach a new house, I would ask the young mother answering the door, "Wouldn't you like for your son to be better off than you are? Wouldn't you want him to be able to have options other than working in the mine? The only way you're going to be able to do this is for him to get a good education, and the way to start that off right is to buy this set of encyclopedias."

Additionally, we sold "The Harvard Classics" originally known as "Dr. Eliot's Five-Foot Book Shelf." It was a fifty-one-volume collection of classic works from world literature, compiled and edited by Dr. Charles Eliot, who had been the president of Harvard University. Eliot had often stated in speeches that the elements of a liberal education could be obtained by spending fifteen minutes a day reading from a collection of books that could fit on a five-foot shelf. The publishing company I worked for at the time, P. F. Collier and Son, saw an opportunity and actually challenged Dr. Eliot to come up with the collection of books for his "shelf." The Harvard Classics was the result. The pitch to the coal mining families was wildly successful, and we ended up selling a lot of books.

The hard work paid off. I was able to support my family, continue to save money to go to medical school while main-

THE SCHOOL YEARS

taining good grades my last year in pre-med. By the time I was ready to apply to medical school, I was in the top 10 percent of my graduating class.

Even though my parents' dream of me graduating from college and being accepted into medical school had now come true, they didn't fully appreciate it. They harped on me, "Why wasn't I number one in my class?" and "Why hadn't I been able to make even more money for my medical school tuition?" This bothered me, but only a little. I had long since learned that I would never please my parents, so why should I even try? My desire to become a doctor now had nothing to do with my parents. My sole goal was to become a physician and please my future patients, guiding them to health, which in those days was more about treating a disease than preventing it.

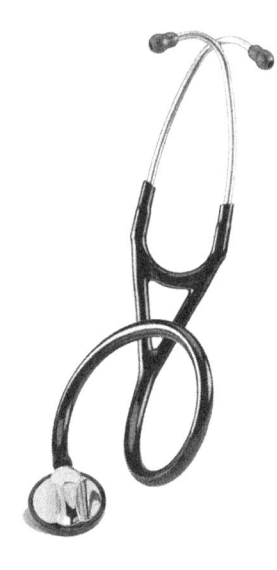

CHAPTER FIVE:

THE INTEGRATIVE APPROACH

While still basking in the glow of graduation from college, I had some important decisions still in front of me. What kind of doctor did I want to be? What kind of medicine did I want to practice?

I realized early on that, for me, it wasn't about "choosing teams" between traditional and alternative approaches to medical practice. It's much more about what is best for the patient. I believe, ultimately, that's what my motivation is all about. That's the thing that drives me most.

There's always been a certain amount of mystery surrounding the alternative approach to medicine but if you think about it, there's mystery surrounding the traditional approaches as well. Let's face it. We know much more than we used to, but there will always be questions. We have so much more to learn.

The Good Doctor

I'm compelled to practice an integrative approach to medicine. For me, it's not about "alternative" or "traditional." It's about whatever it takes to bring healing and relief to the patient. That's the number one priority. It seems so obvious when stated, but you'd be surprised how often, what's best for the patient is not the number one goal.

BONDING WITH THE PATIENT

When I used to teach in medical school, I told the young doctors, "You must bond with the patient!" That was the key from the very first meeting. As doctors, they need to come in with a positive, friendly approach. I taught them to make it a practice to do much more than just find out what's wrong. When you ask about social history, ask whether the patient is on welfare or if they have plenty. Dig in to know all about their socio-economic background and their medical literacy; what is their level of awareness? Are they able to even articulate what's wrong with them? All of this has an enormous bearing on their health and the way we choose to treat them.

I always try to spend a few minutes talking about something other than just medicine or illness. I want to know what interests the patient has. Do they like to go fishing or biking? I try to talk to the patient in their language about the things they care about. I always ask a lot of questions! You never learn if you don't ask questions!

Of course, I always make eye contact, and I do a lot of touching. I believe that there is a tremendous amount of communication that happens nonverbally. In fact, only 7 percent of communication comes from the actual words we speak. Over half

THE INTEGRATIVE APPROACH

of our communication or 55 percent comes from body language and another 38 percent comes from the tone of our voice.

For example, when I speak with a patient complaining of chest pain and ask, "Where is the pain?" I've learned that when they rub their hand up and down the sternum, most of the time it means they are suffering from heartburn. If they point with one finger to an area adjacent to the chest bone, it is costochondritis or arthritis of the rib-sternal joint. On the other hand, if they stretch the right hand over the left chest it is, in almost every case, angina, which is a pain due to the heart muscle not getting enough blood. I've also learned that if they place their fist over the heart it indicates an acute heart attack! So when doctors are busy writing or typing on their laptops or tablets, they could be missing critical clues to a tremendous amount of information.

ALWAYS LOOKING FOR CLUES

Based on clinical experience and original research, Dr. Eric Finzi, in his book, "The Face of Emotion," (2013) shows how changing a person's face not only affects their relationships with others but also brings about changes within themselves. In his studies using Botox, he has shown how inhibiting the frown of clinically depressed patients leads many to experience relief. This work is a dramatic departure from the neuroscience-based thinking on emotions that tends to view emotions solely as the result of neurotransmitters in the brain. A good doctor will be on the alert from the moment he or she encounters the patient. The clues are everywhere!

The Good Doctor

For instance, facial expressions are one of the few remaining body language indicators that humans still have. These expressions are left over from the more common expressions that lower animals still use, a nonverbal display of emotion which signals information to others to either come close or beware! In humans, this constitutes an important, but often overlooked communicative element in social interaction. Whether it was intuition or a gift of God, I discovered this in my practice early on.

Today I actually use a scribe. I have an assistant who comes into the room with me to consult with the patient. This way, I can focus on the patient much more closely.

That's why I take special care with all my patient interactions. The first thing I consider is the room itself. I have done my best to set the patient at ease, even through the design of the room. First of all, I see it not as an exam room…but rather a consultation room, a place for us to talk. In the various rooms in my office, I take care to bring a little different design to each room, setting each apart from the other with separate themes. I've discovered that this serves to entertain the patient while they wait. I take care to leave a generous supply of easy reading medical articles. I also like to make sure each room has good natural light to detect anemia or pale skin better.

A good doctor is like a detective. I probably gain as much by looking at the patient as I do by talking or touching the patient. For instance, I've noticed that in florescent light, you can't see jaundice. Or if the patient comes in with Addison's disease or certain cancers that give a dark hue around the eyes, I can't see this without good natural light in the room.

THE INTEGRATIVE APPROACH

When I initially enter an exam room, with my assistant behind me to take notes, the first thing I do is sit on my roller stool and roll over next to the patient. I like to sit very close, almost knee to knee. Then I'll take the patient's hands in mine. Again, I can tell so much just by touching. I can feel if the hands are cool or warm, dry or moist, shaky or still. These are all indicators of what might be going on in their bodies. At times, I can feel the "vibes" emitting from the patient by sitting close and "feeling them" with my sixth sense.

I'm committed to treating and caring for the patient. One of the most disappointing things I've seen is doctors who put more trust in what the test results say rather than what the patient is telling them. I am fortunate to have learned early on that more times than not, a proper diagnosis came not from the laboratory test but from listening to the patient's health history and being observant during the physical examination. I've always believed that if the laboratory test does not agree with the patient, I choose to throw out the lab report rather than the patient.

All of these things help me bond with the patient. And bonding with the patient helps me overcome what I believe are two of the biggest problems in our health care system today. The first is that doctors today spend, on the average, only about twelve minutes with each patient. Many times the patient isn't even able to see the doctor and is handed off to one of the nurses or physician's assistants. If you've been to see your doctor lately, you know this is true. And often, a lot of that time is spent with the doctor writing or typing and not actually listening, or watching or advising the patient. That's why I do things differently. I want to get to the bottom of what's

The Good Doctor

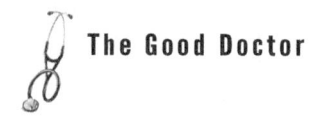

wrong with that patient. And the only way to do that is to spend time with them.

The other big problem with our health care system today is that patients are losing their confidence in their doctor. Patients don't feel like they're heard, and then they are given a prescription or procedure without full explanation of what's happening. It's no wonder they're skeptical.

I know my approach works. I believe in it. But I'm not writing this book so you'll believe in my approach to practicing medicine, although that would be nice. My desire is that you would approach your health care and the health care of your family and loved ones with no blinders on.

Ironically, it's the doctors who seem to be wearing the blinders...not the patients. They've seen the traditional methods practiced in school and are still taught these things in their continuing medical education. They choose to allow this to block their vision for anything else. You would think that all doctors are committed to what's best for the patient. But sadly, that's not the case. Some remain blind to the obvious.

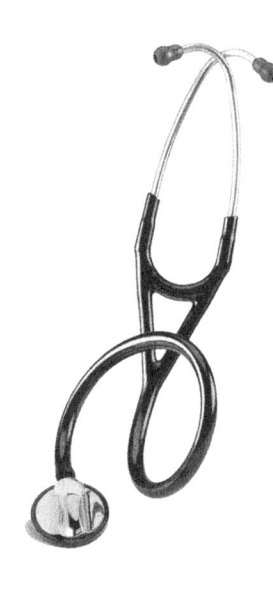

CHAPTER SIX:

THIS I BELIEVE

These truths have caused me to be very intentional about my philosophy of medicine. Ever since people began practicing medicine, they've had to struggle with the "God complex." It's tough to stay humble when you've had years of very sick people coming to you, trusting you, placing their very lives in your hands. It's easy to begin to believe that you do possess some super power that brings healing to all you touch.

While it's true, many doctors have achieved some level of expertise, most doctors, if they are honest, will admit that medicine, healing, and the human body are all still largely a mystery. Most doctors can remember plenty of times when they did everything they knew to be right only to have the patient die anyway. And the converse is also true. There have been times when, in spite of all the wrong assumptions, incorrect diagnoses, and wrong treatments, the patient got better.

At the very center of my belief in medicine is the inalienable right of the patient to have the primary voice in their

The Good Doctor

health care, not the doctor. I believe there is a crippling shortage in the medical practice of physicians who are willing to humble themselves and listen and learn and put the patient and their needs first.

I've had to make some very difficult choices in the arc of my medical career. I've made decisions that have caused my family and me to make great sacrifices. Now looking back, it's easy to see where some of these choices were good and some were not. But each of these decisions was driven by my passion for medicine, and not just medicine alone. I could have poured myself into research. I certainly spent enough time studying. No. What drove me then and continues to drive me to this day is my passion for people and to see them well. I genuinely want to help people. I don't care whether that's through traditional medicine or alternative methods. I want to see patients get well no matter what approach happens to be working.

There's always been a certain amount of mystery surrounding the alternative approach to medicine. I'll admit, those who adhere to the alternative approach are often called quacks. And let's face it, sometimes they can be a pretty strange lot. Some of the treatment plans they believe in do sound pretty weird indeed, especially if you haven't been around these methods.

But if you think about it, there's indeed been mystery surrounding the traditional approaches as well. The truth is, we know much more now than we used to, but there will always be questions in medicine. Always. We have so much left to learn. We will never learn everything there is to know.

THIS I BELIEVE

CHIROPRACTORS ARE DOCTORS TOO

I'm often asked what I think of chiropractors. Sadly, in my early years of medical school I was taught that chiropractors are quacks. But now I've completely changed my mind on that score. The change comes from years and years of experience, of knowing I can't help every patient I see using traditional medical methods. When I was in Sedalia, Missouri, I remember having patients with back problems that I tried to help traditionally only to throw up my hands in surrender. I was humbled to admit there was nothing I could do to help them. I ended up sending them to a chiropractor and watching them get much better and begin to live without pain. That's why I now have no trouble today endorsing chiropractors and the wonderful work they do.

The problem is that doctors who practice traditional methods, by and large have rejected chiropractors and the way they choose to treat their patients. In fact, it used to be illegal for a doctor to even recommend that one of his patients see a chiropractor. Thank God patients are smart enough to go to someone who can help them with their back problems. They wisely consult a chiropractor.

I once wrote an article on EKG's (Electrocardiograms). I wrote about how to administer the test, when it's appropriate to give the test, and what to look for in the results. The article was well received and led to my being able to teach a course on the topic. I was approached by several chiropractors who wanted to take the course. I saw no reason they couldn't take the course and learn what the other doctors were learning. It wasn't long, however, before I got a stern letter from the State Medical Board (in Missouri) telling me that I wasn't allowed to

The Good Doctor

teach the chiropractors in my class. This was my class and my material and yet here I was being told by the State Board whom I could teach and whom I could not teach! That's how strong the prejudices are between these two esteemed methods of practicing medicine.

In 1974, the American Chiropractic Association sued the American Medical Association (AMA) and the American Radiologic Society. I remember traveling to Chicago that year in order to testify on behalf of the chiropractors against the AMA. It was my contention then, and now, that chiropractors should be trained and certified to administer these tests. A patient needing an x-ray or an EKG and not being able to have these tests done by their chiropractor, whom they trust, is unacceptable.

The bottom line for me has always been the patient, what is best for them? As skilled doctors, that should direct us every step of the way in each and every case. Fortunately for the patients, the chiropractors won their lawsuit and could legally begin to become certified to administer CAT scans, mammograms, EKG's and other tests. Up until that time, only MD's could perform those kinds of tests.

Of course in Missouri, where I was practicing at the time, the State Board of Medicine was not too happy with me. They began the process of moving in and looking carefully over my shoulder, watching for the least little excuse to take away my license to practice.

In addition to my traditional medical certifications, I maintained a forty-year membership of the American Academy of Manipulative Doctors. This was an organization of MD's who want to learn the ways that chiropractors have been treating

THIS I BELIEVE

patients for decades. I've been fortunate enough to train MD's in these practices that were long thought to be taboo. The AAMD no longer exists but its influence on me and my practice has shaped me into the kind of doctor I am today.

Going forward, doctors are going to have to work very hard to win back this trust. It's critical. Yes, our current health care system is a mess. Insurance companies have way too much influence on how we practice. Pharmaceutical companies exert too much control. The FDA needs a complete overhaul to get much needed medicines to the market much more quickly. Money, not healing and wellness, has become the primary driver in every step along the way. But it all starts with that magic moment when the doctor and patient come together. Is the number one priority of the doctor and patient and everyone else involved in the healing process all the same thing? Are we all fully committed to seeing that patient get well?

Until this happens, the patient's voice will continue to be largely ignored. Until health care providers are willing to listen and make healing the only priority, I fear we will continue to struggle with mediocrity in the practice of medicine.

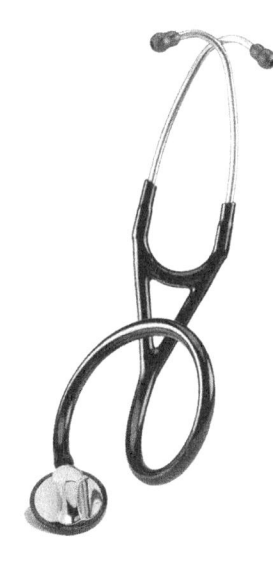

CHAPTER SEVEN:

AN AFFAIR OF THE HEART: THE JOHN TAYLOR STORY

The medical profession has failed John Taylor. Like so many patients, John suffered because of well-meaning doctors who made up their minds too soon. He had to endure a lot of pain and, in the end, an ineffective bypass surgery only because the doctors would not look deeper. John has coronary artery disease.

Coronary artery disease, or simply heart disease, is the number one killer in our country for both men and women. The disease affects over 13 million Americans, and that number is on the rise.

Heart disease is the result of the build-up of unhealthy plaque on the interior lining of the coronary arteries. The

The Good Doctor

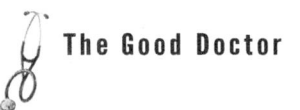

plaque, which is a waxy substance, adheres to the lining of the arteries causing a dangerous restriction of blood flow. The arteries, which start out smooth and elastic, become hard and rigid with the plaque build-up. Ultimately, the heart becomes starved for the oxygen and nutrients the blood delivers. In simple terms, the plaque causes a clogged highway, restricting travel of the blood to the heart.

We know now that John had coronary artery disease. The problem was, he was the only one who suspected it. Try as he might, he couldn't get his doctors to understand how serious his condition was. In fairness to his doctors, John's heart disease was presenting symptoms that looked and sounded a lot like a bad case of acid reflux or heartburn.

It was easy to be fooled. If you were to see John in the mall or on the street, he simply didn't look like a man who suffered from heart disease. Sure, if he smoked two packs a day and was fifty pounds overweight maybe. But John was 180 pounds and 5'11", fully within the normal range for a man his age. So it was hard for his doctors to hear him describe his chest pains and think it was anything but acid reflux.

A DESPERATE CONDITION

But his condition was worsening. Over the coming days and weeks, things would get much more serious for John. In November of 2013, his pain ramped up. He began to suffer from severe chest pains, much worse than before. In fact, the pains were bad enough to send him on a desperate run to the emergency room (ER). The team in the ER did all the tests they knew to do, but there was no sign that John had had a heart attack.

AN AFFAIR OF THE HEART: THE JOHN TAYLOR STORY

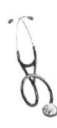

The doctors didn't know what else to do but to send John home. But his chest pains would continue and, unbelievably, they got worse in the coming days. Looking back, John was convinced he was suffering from a series of small heart attacks. The attacks were small enough that they missed the doctor's notice but significant enough to cause John a considerable amount of pain.

John was worried. He was suffering but couldn't seem to find anyone to look deeper than the obvious. He knew he was going to have to go somewhere else to get the answers he needed.

At the time, John worked in a high-stress job. It was on the job that a friend recommended he come see me. My name always seems to come up in these types of situations. Someone shares with a friend about their frustration of not being able to get the answers they need from their traditional doctor and a call to me is recommended.

From his very first visit, John felt assured. Because of the style of my practice, I'm used to taking the time necessary with each and every patient. I remember watching John very closely. I was on the careful lookout for the little subtle things that other doctors had missed. Because I always do my consultations with an assistant in the room to write everything down, I'm not preoccupied writing or typing. I'm able to be more aware of what's happening with the patient.

THE BLOOD KNOWS THE TRUTH

On John's first visit, we did the all important blood test. As noted in another chapter, it's the patient rather than a test that most of the time leads us to a successful diagnosis. It's the

The Good Doctor

doctor's duty to use the test to refute other considerations. In John's case, the tests were ordered to show that, despite his examinations and normal EKGs, something sinister was going on in his body.

The blood test can be, in certain cases, the key that leads the physician to the accurate diagnosis. No matter what the outward, physical findings might be, a critical blood study leads, in most cases, to the correct diagnosis and treatment. Just remember, the blood always knows the truth about exactly what's going on in the body. When I got my hands on the results of John's blood work, an interesting fact jumped out at me.

I told him, "I see here that you can't take statins."

Statins are meds given to those with heart disease to reduce their levels of lipids in the blood. The statins do this by altering the activity in the liver where lipids are produced in the body. Lipids can exacerbate the build-up of plaque.

What I didn't know at the time was that his heart doctor, because of high cholesterol levels, had prescribed John statins. John knew about his high cholesterol because of a wellness test he took at his job, so this was no surprise. He was faithful to take the meds, but they were causing him to suffer miserably. The meds were causing so much joint and muscle pain that John could hardly walk. He had been to see his doctor about the pain, but the doctor didn't make the connection between the statins and the pain. The doctor just told John to continue on the medication.

When I mentioned the results of the blood tests showing no tolerance to statins, a light bulb of recognition went on over John's head.

AN AFFAIR OF THE HEART: THE JOHN TAYLOR STORY

"I knew it! I knew there was something in those meds that was causing me so much pain!"

FRANK'S SIGN

I took another careful look at John. I was sitting close enough to notice a subtle crease in John's earlobe. A normal earlobe is smooth, but an earlobe with a crease has a fold, line, or wrinkle that appears to cut the earlobe in half.

Long ago, in my studies, I read an article in the *New England Journal of Medicine* about this phenomenon. It was about a very interesting study performed by Dr. Sanders T. Frank. Dr. Frank had found that a crease in the earlobe was a potential indicator of heart disease. The crease became known as "Frank's sign."

Although scientists across the country agreed that the link between the disease and the crease existed, they weren't entirely sure how the two were connected. Their only theory is that when the elastic tissue that surrounds the small blood vessels carrying blood to the earlobe becomes more rigid and hard, the telltale crease is formed. Put simply, the visible changes occurring in the tiny blood vessels of the ear (and causing the crease) likely indicate similar changes in the blood vessels around the heart.

Since reading the article, I look carefully for the crease in every patient coming through my office. I saw it now across the room on John's earlobe. Combined with his high cholesterol count and severe chest pains, I was convinced that he didn't have a simple case of heartburn. Even though he didn't

The Good Doctor

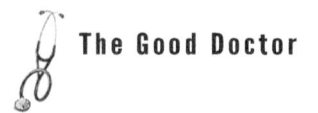

seem a likely candidate, I was certain John had coronary artery disease.

GOOD NEWS...BAD NEWS

I quickly ordered a CAC or Coronary Artery CAT scan. This test was paid for by an insurance study done in the 80s and early 90s. But because of abuse by the medical profession the funding was dropped. Patients now have to pay for this test themselves. Today, even though the test costs less than $100, the prevailing philosophy by both patients and traditionally practicing doctors alike, is that if the insurance doesn't pay for it, no matter how beneficial it might be, it's probably not worth having. While it is true that we overdo tests in this country and yes, most of them are worthless, there are well-conceived studies that show that they can be lifesaving regardless who pays. This was the case with John.

The way it works is that each test is given a score. Typically a score of 400 would give me cause for concern. John's score was an off-the-charts 32,000! I was stunned! After I had taken a moment to compose myself, I was able to present John with an immediate good news/bad news scenario.

The bad news, of course, was that we were able to confirm now that John did have heart disease and a severe case at that. The good news was that he finally had the answers he needed. Now armed with the results of the CAC he could convince any doctor in any hospital or ER of exactly what he needed.

John and his family were scheduled to go to Phoenix for the Christmas holidays that year to see grandchildren. But now, after looking at the results of these tests, John knew that there

AN AFFAIR OF THE HEART: THE JOHN TAYLOR STORY

was no way he wanted to get on a plane in his condition. At my recommendation, John went to the ER immediately.

When John presented the test results to the ER staff, they were convinced that he needed to be admitted. They scheduled him immediately for an angiogram, which is an X-ray test using a special dye and camera to take pictures of the blood flow in an artery.

Sadly, the results of John's test weren't good at all and only confirmed what we knew now to be true. John was very lucky he hadn't already suffered from a "widowmaker," a sudden severe and fatal heart attack. The doctors in the ER found almost total blockage and ordered an immediate triple bypass surgery.

John will testify today that my intuition and willingness to look outside the box, beyond the acid reflux, to find the answers, probably saved his life. John's body type and lifestyle didn't fit the image of someone with heart disease. The traditional medical community failed to pick up on the deeper clues. It was a subtle quarter inch crease in his earlobe that revealed the actual unseen problem.

AND MORE BAD NEWS

But John's problems were not over. In fact, his problem was even worse than he'd originally thought. Although he experienced some short-term relief, less than twelve weeks after the massive triple bypass surgery, John felt the old familiar pain in his chest again. Of course, now he knew that the pains had nothing to do with acid reflux and came in to see me right away.

The Good Doctor

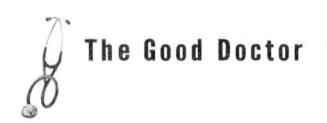

After examining John, I suggested he get back with his heart surgeon as soon as possible to have a deeper look at his problem. On closer inspection, John's doctors found that one of the bypasses had practically disintegrated, and the other two were already entirely blocked again. The unique problem was the clogging was not caused by plaque, which is the normal culprit. John's problem wasn't plaque, and it wasn't scar tissue from the operation.

John's heart doctor told him because of the condition of his arteries the placement of stents was not an option. In many cases, instead of the much more invasive bypass surgery, patients have stents, which is a small expandable tube, inserted into the blocked artery. But John's doctor told him his only choice was more surgery. He wanted to schedule John immediately for a quadruple heart bypass. That would have brought his total number of bypasses up to seven.

With the first surgery now a dismal failure, John was reluctant to go through another ordeal like the first. If there had been some degree of success, it might have been different. But with the blockage returning so quickly, he knew he was going to have to go another way. His doctor told him that if he didn't want the surgery that there was nothing more he could do for him. John chose instead to get a second opinion and came to see me again. He wanted my opinion.

Because I believe in an integrative approach to medicine, I also believe that if traditional medicine doesn't offer satisfactory options, it's time to look carefully at the alternative methods. I recommended that John go on a very strict vegan diet. He now follows the diet described in "Forks Over Knives," a 2011 documentary film that advocates a low-fat,

AN AFFAIR OF THE HEART: THE JOHN TAYLOR STORY

whole foods, plant-based diet. I also encouraged John to take several natural remedies for his condition.

John comes to see me regularly now and views me as his primary care physician. I have become a valuable sounding board for him. He routinely bounces things off me that he hears from his heart specialists. With John's high degree of motivation to get better and my willingness to try new things, we've become a good team, able to achieve some success with John's heart health. He's not out of the woods yet by any means, but he's able to manage his heart health much better now that he knows what's going on. John has come a very long way from the time when he was convinced he wouldn't be around to celebrate his next birthday. In retrospect, we now know John's case much better. He has improved remarkably. His cardiac ejection fraction or EF, which is an indication of his heart function, was in the low 30s and recently it has improved to the 40s (normal is 55 to 60).

John hasn't given up. He didn't only go home and die. He continues to fight. I always look forward to my visits with him. His case has kept me on my toes, always looking for things that might help him—things he can put in his "health care toolbox." Together, we're committed to keep trying to find those things that will work for him.

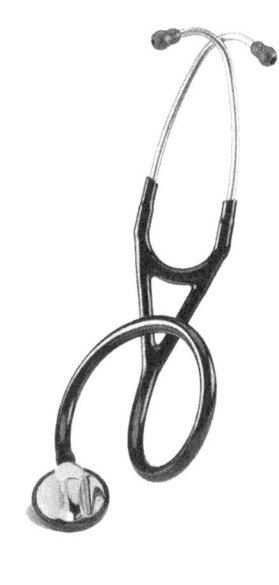

CHAPTER EIGHT:

A DESCENT INTO DARKNESS: KAYE'S STORY

Probably no case in my experience of being a doctor encapsulates my medical philosophy the way Kaye's does. Kaye's case is one of the most dramatic I've ever been a part of. I'm thankful we were able to help her.

A nightmare is a terrifying dream in which the dreamer is overcome by an onslaught of extreme circumstances over which they have no control. In most cases, it's not just one or two negative things, but several events coming at the dreamer at the same time. The anxiety created by this compounding effect can take a toll on the dreamer, even though it's not real.

But what about when the nightmare is real?

The Good Doctor

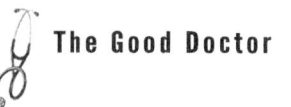

Kaye lived through an ordeal that can only be described as a nightmare. To this day her family is still recovering from the enormous toll that the experience took on them. Her story is one of the strangest, most bizarre I've encountered in my fifty years of practice.

I first met Kaye when she entered my office in May of 2009. From the moment I saw her, it was obvious that this was a tormented woman, a dear soul who had come to the end of her rope. It was apparent she had run out of options and had ended up in my office as a last resort. She'd tried everything else.

Entering the exam room, I sat down on the stool and rolled it up in front of her. Taking her hands in mine, I looked her in the eyes and asked her what was going on in her life. Kaye's desperation told the tale in the lines written across her face. Her story began to spill out, haltingly at first, but then the words tumbled out in a gush.

Kaye was forty-nine years old, and no stranger to physical trials. At birth, she was diagnosed with two heart defects—coarctation of the aorta (a narrowing of the aortic artery) and a hole in one of the chambers of her heart. She underwent her first heart surgery, at five weeks of age, to replace the narrowed portion of her aortic artery. Eighteen years later, in June of 1979, Kaye underwent her second heart surgery in which the previously repaired aortic artery was again replaced. In 1988, at the age of twenty-seven, Kaye was diagnosed with a third heart defect, mitral stenosis, a condition in which the mitral valve is closing. She was told it would only be a matter of time before she would have to undergo yet a third heart surgery to replace the valve. This was devastating news for Kaye and her family.

A DESCENT INTO DARKNESS: KAYE'S STORY

THE ADVENT OF A NIGHTMARE

In July of 2007, Kaye found herself in the ER with a painful ovarian cyst. Twenty years had passed, and her mitral stenosis had not worsened, which baffled her doctors. To avoid further cysts, Kaye was scheduled for a complete hysterectomy. Post-surgery, a dangerous level of fluid built up around Kaye's heart and lungs resulting in congestive heart failure. The compromised mitral valve simply could not pump out the added fluids, and Kaye found herself in a very serious condition. Looking back now, she points to this as the trigger that caused the turmoil that took over her life for the next two years.

Sadly, Kaye is not alone. Adverse side effects are a matter of course with many hysterectomies. My research, in fact, shows that many hysterectomies performed in the U.S. are not needed. Studies show that approximately 90 percent of hysterectomies performed in this country are performed electively, meaning it's up to the patient whether they want the procedure or not. This matches my experience.

Following her hysterectomy, Kaye spent a traumatic five days in the cardiac ICU. She lost approximately ten pounds and felt incredibly weak. For the next few months, she continued to take it easy, being closely monitored by her cardiologist. One evening, Kaye received a late phone call from him. Tests had revealed that the congestive heart failure was still not improving. Kaye's doctor suggested she return to the hospital where she had undergone her 1979 heart surgery, so that doctors there could treat her. As she hung up the phone, suddenly, all those old fears and uncertainties from her youth came flooding back. Would she soon be undergoing yet a third heart surgery? Not only was she suffering physically, but Kaye was also suffering emotionally.

The Good Doctor

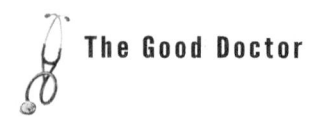

Family members accompanied Kaye on the trip back to the hospital where she had undergone heart surgery some thirty years earlier. Upon arriving at the hospital, the medical staff wasted no time. Kaye was immediately scheduled for several tests, including a heart catheterization. During the tests, the technician reported to Kaye that what had previously been diagnosed as mitral stenosis was actually a third heart defect known as a parachute valve. Instead of opening and closing at full capacity, Kaye's valve was only working at 50 percent capacity. The new diagnosis explained why the condition had not worsened over the years. To Kaye, this was great news. After years of waiting for a valve to completely close, Kaye felt she could finally sit back and take a deep sigh of relief.

After all the tests were run, doctors concluded that in time and with continued medication, Kaye's congestive heart failure would improve. There was no need for another surgery. Kaye's mood began to soar. But even before Kaye left the hospital, family members began noticing a change in her behavior. Serious issues were beginning to line up on Kaye's horizon like the clouds of an Oklahoma summer storm.

A GATHERING STORM

If I had seen Kaye at that time, I could have told her that she was headed for trouble. She was in desperate need of hormone therapy. However, at the time, she had no idea she was in need of anything. She was riding high in the wake of the good news about her heart and returned home on cloud nine, but those feelings weren't to be trusted. In part, they were a lingering effect of a dangerous hormonal imbalance.

A DESCENT INTO DARKNESS: KAYE'S STORY

Kaye's mood swings had become erratic; her emotions were now all over the map. She continued to harbor grandiose ideas and exaggerated emotions...even hallucinations. Feeling that she'd tapped into the fountain of youth, Kaye even hung a poster on her bedroom wall of one of her favorite musical groups from high school. Her energy level soared, and she went from sleeping nine hours at night to only four or five hours. It was as if her brain was on steroids! Ideas were continually flooding her mind; she never felt better, but, around her, her world was beginning to crumble.

Kaye had no clue the effect her strange behavior was having on her family and friends. Anytime one of them would try to talk to her about her bizarre behavior, she discounted their concerns. In her mind, she was the only sane one.

Kaye's euphoria had a flip side. Without warning, she would become volatile, lashing out at those who were closest to her. She was abusive to them and often threatened them with physical harm. To appease those around her, Kaye eventually sought psychiatric help. Although the experts diagnosed her with bipolar disorder, Kaye continued to insist she was just fine.

While the stresses of Kaye's medical condition triggered a mental health issue, there was also a serious hormonal imbalance that needed to be addressed. She was displaying the classic symptoms of someone who desperately needed bioidentical hormone therapy. "Bioidentical" hormones are manmade and they are exactly like the hormones made in the ovaries. The human body can't tell the difference between the two types of hormones. Bioidentical hormones are derived initially from plant sources and are crafted to have the same composition that is naturally produced by the body.

The Good Doctor

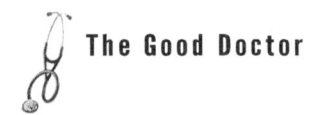

SEARCHING FOR PEACE

By December of 2007, just six months after the hysterectomy, Kaye had morphed into an individual unrecognizable by her loved ones. She was laughing and happy one moment and furious and volatile the next. Ironically, it was around this same time that a terrible ice storm descended upon Kaye's hometown. This destructive storm would shut down this large metropolitan city for days and take the lives of several individuals. Looking back, Kaye would feel that this storm was symbolic of the destruction going on in her own life at that time.

Kaye's story isn't as unique as you might think. Millions of women suffer as their behavior makes them a stranger in their own home. Erratic behavior, combined with the confusion as to the source of the problem, only adds to the hopelessness and despair these women feel.

During this time, Kaye was spending a great deal of time at her parents' home. She found the environment there to have a secure and calming influence on her. It was a familiar place where Kaye could find some peace and she was able to stay there for a while. Her father was someone she refused to fight against and she began to settle down under his influence. This was, perhaps, because when she was growing up, her father demanded respect and obedience from her. Finally, someone was able to get through to her, and Kaye was able to find some peace and relax.

Kaye's faithful husband continued to stay by her side in spite of the erratic emotions that Kaye was displaying nonstop. After all, he had made a commitment twenty-one years earlier to love her for better or for worse; this certainly met the "for worse" criteria. In situations like Kaye's, not only is it difficult for the

A DESCENT INTO DARKNESS: KAYE'S STORY

individual going through the ordeal, it's horrendous for those around her/him too. In Kaye's case, everyone close was suffering.

THE DESCENT INTO DEPRESSION

Around the end of February of 2008, Kaye's emotions began to swing back in the other direction. Her volatility was giving way to an intolerable depression. By now, it had been a roller coaster ride of over six long months, and she was no closer to finding out what the problem was, much less a solution.

As terrible as it was, Kaye's suffering was needless. She was unaware of the many advantages of taking female hormones. Not only does the therapy even out the many severe issues Kaye had to deal with, but it can also do much more. Gynecological problems become markedly improved; uncomfortable and annoying symptoms like hot flashes, night sweats, and mood and sleep disturbances all improve within forty-eight hours of taking female hormones. In Kaye's case, hormone therapy could have halted the problem before it got any worse. Sadly, Kaye's roller-coaster ride had a ways to go before she would find me, and a solution to her mounting problems.

By now, depression had become Kaye's constant companion. Unable to get up in the morning, she was forced to quit her job. The depression was becoming a weight she could hardly bear. Although she wasn't, Kaye felt completely alone and isolated. That isolation cast over her an unrelenting cloud of darkness. The pain was unbearable. Who had she become? She had become estranged from the person she once had been. Kaye's feelings of guilt and loss were too difficult for her to bear.

The Good Doctor

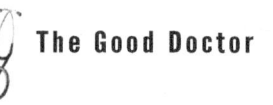

Going to a local mental health hospital for intense and sometimes even in-patient counseling, Kaye fought the depression, but it was getting no better. She was taking Xanax to help curb her anxiety and Ambien to help her sleep. Only when she was sleeping could Kaye find peace, so she began staying in bed for days at a time. Now she had the medication that provided the escape she so desperately needed. She was self-medicating to the point that she could no longer care for herself. Kaye retreated to bed, where she would stay for the next seven months.

Female hormones and their cycle are no mystery for modern medicine. Doctors willing to provide this treatment find success in the battle of balance in their patients' lives. The hormones typically are given by a patch, creams, or pellet.

The cream or gels are not my favorite since the active compounds are absorbed erratically. I'm not a fan of the patches because there are no marketed patches that contain *both* estrogen *and* testosterone. For the last twelve years I have favored the pellet, which is the size of a grain of rice and is inserted under the skin in a sterile and painless procedure taking five minutes. The hormones last about six months and the out-of-pocket expense is about $350, the same as the cream and less than a prescribed branded hormone. Also, the pellet is much more physiologic.

We humans have circulating in our blood SHBG (serum hormone binding globulin), which naturally increases at times of exercise, sex, and stress. The active hormone is released from the pellet as it is needed. Moreover, the SHBG reflects our natural bio-circadian rhythm with the innate early morning rise of the sex and adrenal hormones. The more SHBG is released, the more the hormone is taken out of the pellet. It is

A DESCENT INTO DARKNESS: KAYE'S STORY

like having a bio-implant of a real ovary and adrenal gland! The adrenal gland also releases these hormones while the lady is young and healthy but to a lesser amount in a stressed older woman like Kaye.

An added bonus of having the pellet installed is that it "cures" migraines. It is the sudden decrease in estrogen that triggers many of these headaches. This is why migraines are more common in women compared to men and that they are more frequent right before menstruation.

I recommend progesterone be taken orally versus injection. Not only does taking this oral natural hormone application do all the good things that happen in the injections, it also protects the breast and uterus, while safeguarding the brain. When taken orally and absorbed through the intestine, progesterone is converted in the liver to Allopregnanolone. Also known as Nootripic, it is referred to as a smart drug, with memory, neuro, cognitive, and intelligence enhancer abilities. This hormone actually protects the brain from insult such as free radical damage caused by her environment including stress. Moreover, this has been shown to heal the nervous tissue itself and is now being researched for Alzheimer's and the treatment of spinal cord/brain injury. In a recent study, for cardiovascular health it was statistically significant in good cholesterol and showed some improvement in coagulation, inflammation, blood pressure, weight, and endothelial health.

A DEADLY SCHEME

Gradually, Kaye's depression led to thoughts of suicide. She was obsessed day and night with thoughts of how she

The Good Doctor

might end her life. A plan, fuzzy at first but then more detailed, began to take shape in her mind. First, she would need to get her hands on her meds; they were key to her suicidal strategy. Sensing Kaye's vulnerability, her family put her medications away in a lock box so Kaye could not access them on her own.

The first stage of the plan was to write to her husband a suicide note to explain her desperation and to say good-bye to those she loved. Trying to make some sense out of the craziness of the past months, Kaye explained that she could no longer live as a prisoner of her own mind. Apologizing for her weakness, Kaye instructed her husband where he could find her body the next morning. After typing and printing the letter, Kaye slipped it into an envelope. She got up out of bed and quickly dressed. Then she waited for her opportunity to act.

It was dusk when Kaye realized those around her were distracted. After silently grabbing the lock box with the meds and placing it in a box, Kaye snuck out of the house before anyone realized she was gone. She wanted to put her note in an obvious place but not a place her family would find too soon. So she went around to the backyard and taped the suicide note to the back door, knowing that her family would see it when they checked on the dogs. Then, getting into her car, she drove away, convinced that her decision was the right one.

Kaye's first stop was a hardware store where she had someone help her pry the lock box open. Now that she had access to the meds, her plan was coming together. She drove to a nearby hotel and checked into a room. The weight of the pain was unbearable. She looked forward to the emptiness that eternal sleep would bring. Taking a deep breath, Kaye downed

A DESCENT INTO DARKNESS: KAYE'S STORY

forty Xanax and forty Ambien with huge gulps of water. Then she lay back on the bed to await the peace she knew would come. Finally, her suffering was coming to an end.

After realizing that Kaye had vanished, her husband notified the police about the developing situation. He quickly got in his car and spent the next six hours driving around to hotels and various locations looking for his wife. Exhausted physically and mentally, he returned home sometime after midnight. He began to pray for help and direction. Suddenly, the dogs in the backyard began to bark and wouldn't stop. To this day, Kaye and her husband both believe that God was at work, prompting the dogs to cause a commotion to get her husband to the back door. Opening the back door, he saw the note and immediately called 911. The paramedics instructed him to meet them at the hotel Kaye mentioned in the note. Arriving moments later, they burst into the room to find Kaye on the bed and in a very deep sleep.

Immediately, the paramedics loaded her on a gurney and began pouring liquid charcoal down her throat. The liquid charcoal, also called activated charcoal, absorbs the drugs and neutralizes their effects. The next day, Kaye awoke in the hospital confused and overcome with disappointment. She was still alive and so was the depression and pain. Her much thought-out plan had failed and Kaye was furious with her husband for having saved her life. All those problems and all that pain that she thought she was leaving behind were hovering in the room with her. The torment was horrible, so horrible in fact that she didn't even want to be awake. She longed for the peace that comes with slipping away forever. She prayed, "God, please take my life or let me take it." Now, the grief of

The Good Doctor

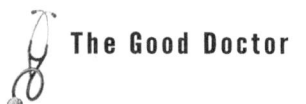

her failure was added as a new layer to her pain. After a few more days in the hospital, Kaye was released to the care of her family.

Concerned for Kaye's safety, her family took her to one of the most prestigious mental health hospitals in the country. She spent five months there in constant therapy of one kind or another. She endured electro-shock therapy three times a week for five weeks.

Meanwhile back in Tulsa, life was passing her by. Kaye's much beloved father was dying. She was able to travel home from the hospital in order to be by his side when he passed. How much more could she take? Like an endless stretch of highway, her pain continued with no end in sight. Returning to the mental health hospital without much hope, she endured another three long months of therapy. In March, she returned home, still severely depressed and still thinking constantly about escaping the pain through suicide.

THE DAWN OF A NEW DAY

That's when her sister happened to watch the Oprah show on television. On the program, Oprah's guest spoke about the successes many women were having with bio-identical hormone therapy. The message got through. Kaye's sister thought, *Could this be the key for Kaye?* With a little investigation, she found that I was the only doctor in Tulsa who administered this kind of treatment.

Kaye's appointment was made, and she came to see me in May of 2009, now almost two long years after her nightmare began. I spent over two hours with Kaye on that first visit.

A DESCENT INTO DARKNESS: KAYE'S STORY

From the moment I met her, I could tell by reading her face that she had been through a horrific ordeal. I did all I could to assure her that we, together, would get to the bottom of the mystery surrounding her health.

After a careful examination and interview, I ordered blood work and told Kaye I'd have the results back in seven days. She was so depressed that this news did little to brighten her mood. In fact, she told me she might not even be alive in seven days. She'd been driven to the end of her rope, and I knew that asking her to wait seven days for the results before treating her was going to be too long. I decided to do what I've done so many times before. I trusted my gut. Instead of waiting, I gave her the first dosage of hormone therapy. I took her hands in mine, looked her in the face, and with as much human compassion as I could muster, I told her to hold on…relief was coming. Just give it time.

By the time the seven days had passed, she was completely symptom-free. The change was gradual, but, by the end of a week, she knew that the cloud had lifted. No more depression. Kaye couldn't believe it. The pellet and the hormones it contained brought the much needed relief and balance to Kaye's life and emotions.

Kaye's tragic story has a happy ending for which I'm grateful. As her doctor, it grieves me that she had to endure so much. It didn't have to be that way. Unfortunately, I see far too many women with similar stories, maybe not to the extent or severity, but traumatic to the patient nonetheless. The fact is that too many women in our country are not taking hormones simply because of the false concern that they might cause cancer.

The Good Doctor

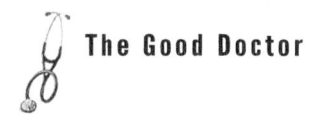

MISGUIDED DIRECTION

Many doctors were hoodwinked back in 2006 when the media began to publish reports that found that taking hormones could be risky. The doctors were willing to believe the reports even though they contradicted over forty years of success in over 1,000 studies.

Today, a woman who is age fifty and in otherwise good health could very well spend half her lifetime in a postmenopausal hormone imbalance. The worst-case scenario is that she could end up much like Kaye. It's troubling to imagine that these women would suffer from something that's so easily treated. Female hormones are the only hormone abnormality in all of medicine that's not routinely replaced. If the patient is found to have a low thyroid level, the doctor will prescribe thyroid. If she has low parathyroid, the doctor will give her parathormone, and no physician would dare withhold insulin from a diabetic. But many physicians are not giving female hormones to those who need it most. Recent statistics show that less than 20 percent of postmenopausal women receive hormonal replacement, and I'm sure many of these women are begging their doctors to prescribe them.

When Kaye came into my office, she wasn't just a number, or a customer, or just a patient with a file and medical insurance. She was a friend, a friend who desperately needed help. I'm just glad I knew what to do. Now, Kaye is on the other side of her terrible nightmare. She's turned the corner, and she's never felt better!

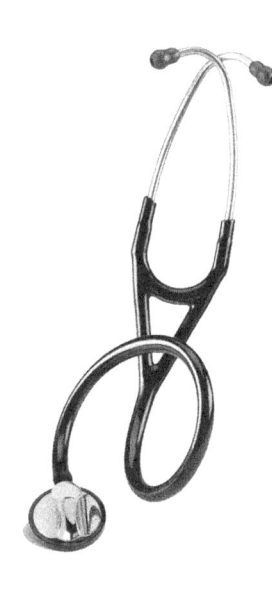

CHAPTER NINE:

MEDICAL SCHOOL

Have you ever had a dream come true? Have you yearned for something with all your heart and soul and finally after many years and many prayers seen it come to pass? If so, then you'll know there's no feeling in the world quite like watching a dream start to become a reality.

My original plan was to attend med school with Chucky. We were looking forward to continuing the tradition of going to school together. Chucky's father had gone to the University of Pennsylvania for three years before going to Jefferson Medical College. Chucky had enrolled as a pre-dental student at Pennsylvania but then transferred over to Muhlenberg, who at the time had a great reputation for getting their graduates into medical school. Chucky had switched to pre-med and done well; he had already been accepted to Jefferson. I applied and might have been accepted there too.

The Good Doctor

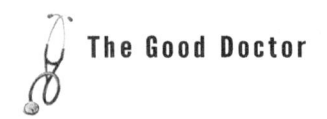

MR. BLOCK, WHY DO YOU WANT TO BE A DOCTOR?

One school I was particularly interested in hearing from was the Seaton Hall Medical School, which later became the New Jersey College of Medicine. Until 1956, they hadn't been a fully accredited medical college because of an arcane law on the books called the Anti-Vivisection Law. This law prohibited medical students from operating on live human patients. Finally in 1956, this law was repealed, paving the way for the medical school to eventually become fully accredited and certified. In 1961, NJCM became a part of Rutgers University.

It was with mixed emotions that I received the news that NJCM wanted to interview me. I was thrilled to get the interview but at the same time, I was terrified. It's one thing to fill out an application and maybe write an essay or two, but it's quite another thing to sit in front of a panel of doctors and educators who will decide your fate based on your responses to their questions. I knew I needed to represent myself well. I would have to exude confidence I didn't feel. I would have to do it in a way that would convince the panel that I was worthy of admittance into their prestigious medical school. I grew up selling newspapers in the rough and tumble world of Atlantic City's back streets and famous Boardwalk. I knew how to handle myself, but this was entirely different. What I needed wasn't brashness and boldness; it was polish and panache. I knew Chucky could help me prepare.

I mustered my courage and told Chucky all about my predicament. He was disappointed that I wanted to go to a different school, but just like so many times before he stepped up to coach me through. He told me exactly the things I should talk about, but more importantly, he told me when to keep my mouth shut. "Don't answer a question they're not asking!" he instructed.

I still remember the man on the panel looking at me over the top of his horn-rimmed glasses. With a stern look meant to intimidate, he asked, "Mr. Block, why do you want to become a physician?" That was the easiest question of the day; it was the moment I had been waiting for. I didn't need coaching to answer this one! I had dreamed of becoming a doctor since I was seven years old. All that hard work, all those long hours working with my father, and later all those hot days walking the beach fully dressed carrying a seventy-five pound box on my back for hours on end. Getting up at 4 a.m. to be first to get the best corner on the Atlantic City Boardwalk to hawk the latest papers, all those late nights staying up studying…it all boiled down to this one question. I had the answer. I cleared my throat, sat up straight, and spoke from my heart, "I want to help people. I want to be in a position where I can help others." Even though I felt very positive about my interview, the faces of the panel were noncommittal as I left the room. I steeled myself for the long wait to hear if I'd been accepted or not.

As I anxiously waited to hear, fear and insecurity began to creep in on the edges of my mind. I had to work hard to keep my vivid imagination in check. Was I good enough to go to school by myself…without Chucky there to help me? Would I ever hear from another school? Was this going to be the end of my quest to become a doctor?

As it turned out, I only had to wait a couple of weeks.

The Good Doctor

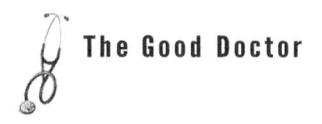

THE HAPPIEST DAY OF MY LIFE

I still remember the day it happened. While my top choice was still Seton Hall, I hadn't given up hope that I might hear from Jefferson Medical School. I approached the mailbox and took a deep breath before reaching in and finding a thick envelope. It was from the Seton Hall Medical School. My hands were shaking with so much excitement that I could barely open the envelope. I tried to rip it open neatly but with my shaking hands, I practically destroyed the envelope just attempting to get it open. With all my heart I wanted to know what was in that letter but I couldn't bear to read the words, "We regret to inform you...." But as it turned out, my fears were unfounded.

I had received an early acceptance! But it was conditional. I had to let them know within two weeks or they would put me into the mix of several thousand other candidates. In those years, less than 10 percent of legitimate medical school candidates that apply were ever accepted. Additionally, I was going to have to send a picture and state my religious affiliation. I was Jewish and most schools at that time had a quota of what percentage of Jewish students they would accept. Seton Hall was a Jesuit School and anti-Semitism in the early 1960s was rampant on the East coast. While not published, I was able to find out later that their quota of Jewish students was only 10 percent.

I was in a daze. On the way back to my apartment, I had to read the opening sentence of the letter several times to be sure it was really true. The letter began, "Congratulations!" I don't even remember what the rest of the letter said. I was so thrilled. It was actually happening...I was taking another critical step toward becoming a doctor. I had been accepted into medical school. That was the happiest day of my life.

MEDICAL SCHOOL

I thanked God then and every day of my life since for allowing me to go to medical school and to become the person I have dreamed of since I was seven years old. I was still waiting for other possible acceptance letters but I believed in the old adage, "one in the hand is worth two in the bush." So I sent my consent to their acceptance and decided not to wait for the Jefferson Medical School acceptance that may or may not have come.

THE MONEY CHALLENGE

When I started medical school, I had to face some harsh realities. Being accepted into Seton Hall wasn't the same as having the money to pay for it. I already knew I couldn't ask my parents for financial assistance. They made it abundantly clear from the start. They admired my dream of becoming a doctor, but they wouldn't be able to help me financially achieve that dream. I was going to have to work at outside jobs to put myself through med school and support my young family.

Early in my first year of medical school, I hauled my snowball cart the 130 miles to Jersey City. When the weather was warm, I sold snowballs. But when the days turned cooler, I sold encyclopedias in various neighborhoods around New Jersey. By then the work had almost become a hoax, and I felt like it was telling a falsehood. We were charged to go door-to-door giving the pitch: "We will give you a set of encyclopedias free if you agree to buy the Yearbook (which was a hardbound year-in-review book) for the next ten years." They also had to agree to write a letter of recommendation that we could use, telling us that the encyclopedias were what they expected and had yielded the desired results in their family. We would then use those letters to make further sales in that area.

I quickly realized I was not being truthful with these poor folks who were just scraping by. The Yearbook cost $39 or more a year for ten years which was over $400! If they chose to pay it off in two years, they would get a beautiful bookcase and the Junior Classics, which was the children's edition of the Harvard Classics. I was heartsick. As a physician, I had pledged to be ethical. "Selling" encyclopedias under these false pretenses had no integrity, and I couldn't be a party to it.

When summer rolled back around, I stayed with what had worked before and went back to Atlantic City to sell snowballs. When I returned to school in Jersey City, I took my cart back with me and sold the snowballs there too.

The snowballs sold well as long as the weather was hot. But when the days turned cool and then cold, I had to figure out a way to supplement my income without going back to selling encyclopedias. This was in the days before student loans, and there was almost no way a broke student like me was going to be able to borrow money for school. Many of my peers were going to school on the GI bill, with their tuition and even room and board paid for, but I wasn't able to take advantage of those benefits.

GOING TO SCHOOL DEBT-FREE

I started washing laboratory glassware every day after class. I'd stay until late at night when I would finally go home to study. In addition to cleaning the glassware, there was a kind professor of cardiology who allowed me to assist him with

MEDICAL SCHOOL

his research, which I could do at home. The research involved reading EKG and cardiac catheterization printouts, then calculating the results. I also became a laboratory technician at a nearby hospital and even received a little scholarship assistance for academic achievement. Again, I was not afraid to put in the hours to work hard! As a result, my family and I made it through all of college and medical school without owing a cent to anyone, including friends, relatives, and even my parents! We did it!

As the weeks counted down for me to go to Jersey City to begin medical school, I decided to arrive a couple of weeks early in order to get an apartment and work on other details to get my family settled before the press of school began.

BUCKLING DOWN, STUDYING HARD

The first two years of medical school are called Basic Science. That meant I had to take courses in Anatomy, Physiology, Bacteriology, and other core science classes. Here I was, chomping at the bit to see actual patients but having to buckle down and study hard to pass these classes. In my youthful zeal, it seemed that these classes had very little to do with the real practice of medicine. This made a big difference in my continuing medical education. I realized that I could think for myself without being beholden to the "greats" to give me what they thought was Medical Truth. I could broaden my thinking, choosing to refute what they had to say or I could choose to accept it and even add on to the things they were teaching. But ultimately, I knew I was going to have to do well in these preliminary courses or I'd be stopped in my tracks before seeing a single patient.

The Good Doctor

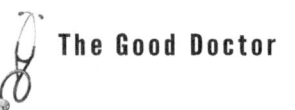

The study habits I'd learned from Chucky once again gave me a leg up. I was able to do well in these core science classes because of my ability to memorize pages and pages of difficult content. Like Anatomy, for instance, I remembered every nerve and every little blood vessel. I memorized where the vessels traveled throughout the body. I learned the muscles, the origin and the exertion, the action. I committed it all to memory. And once again, thanks to Chucky's study tips, I did quite well.

I still remember the first day we started in the Anatomy Lab. It was "odoriferous" to say the least! But I didn't mind the smell at all. I was beginning to feel more and more like a real doctor every day! I was a med school student and was on my way!

Our professor led us into an extremely aromatic room that none of us liked much. It was cold and I was glad for the extra layer of my new white doctor's coat! Even though the room smelled terrible, it gleamed brightly. The tables, the instruments, the lighting...everything in the room was brand new. I was overcome with the sense of gratitude just standing there.

I remember that first day...my team named our cadaver "Eddie." Before starting our procedures each day, we thanked God for Eddie and his willingness to give his body so that we might learn how to help other people.

Even though there are many more campuses now, at that time there was only one campus and that was in Jersey City. At the time of its founding, Franklin Roosevelt actually came to lay the cornerstone. It was the largest facility in New Jersey with close to 3,000 beds.

MEDICAL SCHOOL

In that first year's class there were about 115 students. Seton Hall was established under the auspices of the Roman Catholic Archdiocese of Newark, so it was no surprise that the majority of students accepted each year were Catholic. However, the admissions committee had heard that Jewish students make good doctors and, as I mentioned earlier, had established a quota for Jewish students. At the time, I was a practicing Jew, not an overly zealous one, but I was proud of my heritage and did nothing to hide the fact from my mostly Catholic colleagues.

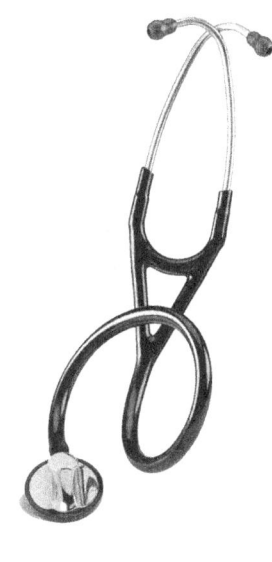

CHAPTER TEN:

COMPOUNDING ISSUES: CRYSTAL'S STORY

In 1994 Crystal's life was a mess. She'd seen several doctors and had been diagnosed with a whole host of serious medical conditions like fibromyalgia, carpal tunnel syndrome, and severe arthritis. She suffered from other symptoms as well—mysterious symptoms difficult for the doctors to categorize and diagnose.

Crystal was like many of the patients I see every week. She'd seen many doctors over the years and spent lots of money trying to find answers with no luck. The mystery and confusion surrounding her condition only made her pain greater.

When one specialist suggested surgery for her carpal tunnel syndrome, she had a brief moment of hope. "Maybe this operation would take away my constant pain," she thought. Perhaps this procedure would make me feel healthy again. She hoped that this surgery would be the end of her troubles but that hope was short-lived. The doctor told her that although he does many of these surgeries, almost 80 percent of them are not successful. Ultimately, in most cases, the operations bring no relief from the pain of carpal tunnel.

Crystal was heartbroken. There was no way she wanted to endure the additional pain of surgery on top of the pain of the carpal tunnel, especially when the outcome offered such a slim hope of success. She went with her gut and declined the doctor's recommendation of surgery.

Crystal's health issues worsened and now even threatened her livelihood. She loved her job and got to interact with lots of different people. But she had a huge territory to cover and spent a lot of time in her car. On the average, she drove over 2,500 miles every month. Her pain had become so great she could no longer endure the long hours sitting in the car.

ADRIFT IN PAIN

With the causes of her various ailments still such a mystery, Crystal was lost with no idea what to do. And because she had no plan, her condition continued to worsen. By 2004, ten years after the original diagnoses, her weight had ballooned to over 235 pounds. Her pain was so debilitating that she spent most of her days on the couch doing her best to mask the pain by eating things that only made things worse. She was tempted to give up.

COMPOUNDING ISSUES: CRYSTAL'S STORY

But Crystal wasn't raised to give up. She was raised on the prairie and married to a cowboy. She knew all about hard work, and she was used to life dealing difficult hands. She had learned to be a fighter, a finisher. It was this stubborn frontier spirit that kept her from completely giving up.

She decided to harness her courage to make another circuit through the medical profession in search of answers. One doctor, after many rounds of expensive blood tests, diagnosed lupus. Lupus is an autoimmune disease where the body's immune system becomes hyperactive and attacks normal, healthy tissue. This can result in symptoms such as inflammation and swelling, and can cause damage to joints, skin, kidneys, blood, the heart, and lungs. The symptoms were close to Crystal's and she thought this could be the answer. But then came the bad news that there's no medical cure for lupus and there hasn't been a new drug to treat the disease in over fifty years.

Crystal was disappointed when the doctor's only recommendation was for her to lose some weight. Crystal thought, "Is that all he could do for me? After spending all that money on all those tests, I thought he'd be able to tell me something I didn't already know!" Crystal's cries for help were falling on deaf ears.

DECIDING TOO QUICKLY

This actually happens more than you might think. As in the earlier case of John Taylor, doctors often make up their minds too quickly as to the problem with the patient sitting in front of them. They rely too heavily on the results of tests

The Good Doctor

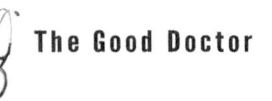

instead of relying on a close examination of their patient. Listening to the patient should always be an important part of the analysis process. As I've mentioned, my adage for practice has always been to trust what the patient tells me over what the report tells me.

The misinformation and missed diagnoses continued to plague Crystal. Another doctor, this one an OB/GYN, ran some tests and told Crystal she was "full of cancer". He recommended an immediate D and C, a surgical procedure that involves the removal of part of the lining of the uterus by scraping it off. Once again, this diagnosis seemed off to Crystal. She continued her search. She saw an endocrinologist and a rheumatologist, but no one had the answers she sought. It seemed her condition had everyone stumped.

There was one thing all the experts could agree on. Even Crystal knew her body well enough to read the obvious signs; every one of the critical systems of her body was completely out of control. It was as if her body was attacking itself. She was scared. Could there be anything worse than your body working against you? Crystal found herself at the end of her rope. She was desperate for a solution that would finally give her some relief from the torment she was living through.

AND THEN ONE DAY

And then one day...

Don't so many of our life stories begin to turn on that simple four-word phrase? And then one day, Crystal was on her couch, as usual, listening to the radio. She was depressed. The dark clouds of confusion had descended and enveloped

COMPOUNDING ISSUES: CRYSTAL'S STORY

her. She was in pain and could find no promise of relief. Even her fierce stubbornness had left, and she no longer had the strength nor the will to fight.

Crystal was frustrated with her health, with her weight gain and with the fact that she'd allowed herself to become trapped on her couch. She was frustrated at what her life had become and that she couldn't find the answers to make it better. She was even frustrated with what was playing on the radio. She reached over and gave the dial a halfhearted turn, not caring where it landed.

That's when Crystal found me. The dial stopped at a station carrying my "All Things Medical" radio program. The dial stopped at the exact moment I was reading a list of conditions I was busy treating in many of the patients I was currently seeing. My list looked just like her list: fibromyalgia, carpal tunnel syndrome, and severe arthritis. These were all ailments a colleague and I were successfully treating.

Needless to say, I now had Crystal's full attention. She sat up on the couch and immediately began to look for a pen and paper to take down my contact information. At the time, I was offering to see uninsured patients for only $50. After the exorbitant amounts Crystal had been used to paying to other doctors she could hardly believe her ears. Could her solution be waiting in a simple doctor's office in Coffeyville, Kansas, for only $50? Now she just had to convince her husband Earl to spend more hard-earned money, just one more time, in the hopes they would finally find some answers.

Earl was only too happy to spend the money if the appointment would promise hope for his wife. Crystal called and made an appointment. On the day of the scheduled visit, she

The Good Doctor

carefully gathered the collection of papers that detailed her baffling medical history over the last ten years. She clung to the file hoping that I could find the answer to the mystery buried somewhere in those papers. She carried the file in front of her like a shield as she entered the exam room and waited to be seen.

SEEING A NATUROPATH

My colleague was scheduled to see her and confidently walked into the exam room and immediately saw the thick file in her lap. Crystal was shocked at his first words to her. "I don't need to see your file. Just sit down here and I'll tell you what's wrong with you."

That was certainly unexpected! Here was someone who not only offered a solution, but also offered it without even looking at her medical history. Crystal was skeptical but allowed herself a glimmer of hope.

The practitioner took the time to listen to Crystal and do a careful examination. He ordered some strength testing and was able to quickly rule out the earlier diagnosis of lupus. Next, a few simple blood tests revealed Lyme disease and some problems with her thyroid gland. This was all news to Crystal. None of these issues had even come up at any of her doctor visits over the previous ten years. She finally had names to put with the mysterious enemies attacking her body.

Crystal left our offices that day with a bag full of supplements, a list of foods to avoid, and something else; she had a renewed sense of hope. From that day forward, Crystal started getting better. Under our care, Crystal's improvement was

COMPOUNDING ISSUES: CRYSTAL'S STORY

dramatic. The symptoms that had plagued her for many years began to disappear. She was able to lose weight. She was able to sleep through the night again.

BRALY'S SIGN

Crystal's improvement was an enormous encouragement for her. But I noticed something else. On one of her visits, I asked to look closely at Crystal's hands. She held them out for me, and I noticed that her pinkie finger was just a little shorter than the last joint of her ring finger. This is a common telltale indicator of gluten intolerance known as Braly's sign. While this observable diagnosis was discovered in Poland in 1953, it didn't catch on in this country until popularized by the English expert James Braly, MD.

Because of this, I had a hunch that along with everything else she had been suffering from, Crystal was also gluten intolerant. Gluten intolerance or its more serious condition, Celiac disease, is vastly underdiagnosed. It takes an average of eleven years between the first appearances of bowel symptoms and the time it's finally correctly diagnosed.

Gluten is the most common significant allergen known to civilized man. It's a protein, which is frequently found in wheat. It's estimated that 10 percent of the population are sensitive enough to gluten to be considered gluten intolerant. In addition to wheat, gluten can also be found in rye, spelt, triticale, and kamut. Although not all doctors agree, gluten may also be found in dark beans, oats, and peanuts. Non-gluten cereals are rice, millet, tapioca, buckwheat, flaxseed, teff, and quinoa

The Good Doctor

(keen-wa). Gluten is not found in vegetables and meat, but it is used in 90 percent of all protein-fortified products.

REMEMBER B-R-O-W-S FOR GLUTEN

We had quite a list of dietary recommendations for Crystal when she left that day! I told Crystal, and I tell others with this condition, to stay away from B-R-O-W-S: where B stands for Barley and Beans (green), R for Rye, O for Oats, W for Wheat, and S for Spelt.

Crystal was confident that she was on the right track. I encouraged her to make the life-changing decision to stay away from BROWS and she readily agreed. Her improvement accelerated.

Today, though we've moved our office from Coffeyville to Tulsa, Crystal continues to come a few times a year for treatment. She willingly drives the 180 miles (one way). Crystal is now my patient, and I'm blessed to have her.

Crystal says, "It was clear I was dying. No one could tell me what was going on in my body until I met with that naturopath. And now, I'm so blessed to have found Dr. Block. I drive the miles to see him because I know he's the right doctor for me. He's a teaching doctor who believes that the patient knows best about what's going on in their body. Dr. Block expects me to be a student of the things that are happening with me. I know I'm in charge of my own treatment, and I like that. It's empowering after years of dealing with doctors who believed differently. I've never known a doctor like Dr. Block. I'm thankful for him!"

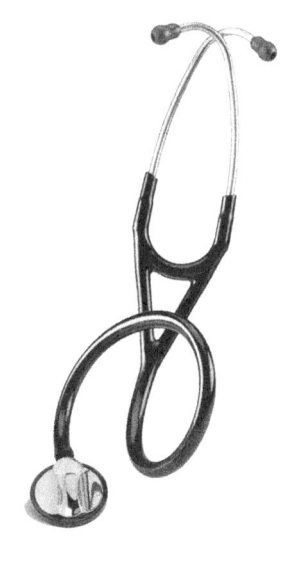

CHAPTER ELEVEN:

A ROSE BY ANY OTHER NAME IS STILL A ROSE: ROSE'S STORY

For much of my practice, I've known that many of my patients are coming to me as the last resort. It's not odd at all to have a patient come and see me only after spending many years and many thousands of dollars under the care of other doctors all to no avail.

I think it's fair to say many of my patients are desperate. They've gotten their hopes up so many times only to be crushed when no answers came. They've come to the end of their rope. It's one thing to be sick, to know that something is not right in your body. Add to that the confusion and helplessness of not

The Good Doctor

being able to find the answers you need, and you've got a recipe for desperation.

If there's one thing I've noticed over the years of my practice, it's the importance of hope in the healing process. In many cases, if the patient has hope, they can overcome even the direst of situations. I've seen patients overcome a multitude of serious issues with only hope to grab ahold of. On the other hand, I've seen patients lose ground and go down hill quickly and ultimately die when they could've lived, all because they'd given up hope. I maintain that hope is the most important medicine a person can have in their medical toolkit.

It was that way with Rose. She never gave up hope. And she had plenty of opportunities to do just that. She came to me several years ago after being referred to me by my friend and colleague.

Rose was diagnosed with several inflammatory diseases like rheumatoid arthritis, Crohn's disease, and lupus. She had been diagnosed by her regular group of doctors practicing the traditional approach. She was on several prescription medications, but they weren't helping her condition. She was taking a handful of pain medications as well to help her deal with the pain. She was in such bad shape she couldn't get out of bed in the morning.

She knew of my colleague, a naturopath, because she worked in an adjoining office space. She had resisted going to see him because she was still convinced the answer lie with the more traditional methods. It wasn't until the traditional doctors prescribed a Remicaid IV drip that she first began to open up to the idea of finding another way of healing. Rose was concerned that the Remicaid would eventually destroy her

A ROSE BY ANY OTHER NAME IS STILL A ROSE: ROSE'S STORY

body's immune system, and she began her search for alternatives. It was her husband Tom who first encouraged Rose to seek alternative treatment. She resisted at first but after much pleading, Rose reluctantly agreed. She told her husband that she would try the alternative route for thirty days. She called and made an appointment.

THE PATIENT BECOMES THE STUDENT

Over the years of illness, Rose had learned to become a student of her body. She probed the Internet looking for answers. She knew that there must be answers out there somewhere. The more research she did, the more she actually looked forward to her visit with her doctor if for no other reason than to hear a different perspective.

She wasn't sure what to expect, but whatever it was, it wasn't what she got. From her first impression, she found the doctor to be abrupt and opinionated. But eventually, his confidence in his own answers began to reassure Rose. His confidence caused Rose's confidence in his ability to grow. After so many doctors shrugging their shoulders and giving up, it was nice to have a doctor who thought he knew the solution to her many medical issues.

In that very first visit, he agreed with the findings of the traditional doctors that she was indeed suffering from the inflammatory diseases, rheumatoid arthritis, Crohn's disease, and lupus. But he found something else, Lyme disease. Lyme disease is the most common tick-borne disease in the northern hemisphere. Early symptoms may include high fever, headache, and fatigue. If left untreated, the symptoms can spread to involve the joints, the heart, and even the central nervous system. These symptoms were familiar to Rose, but all the other things she was dealing with at the time were masking them.

She was instructed to remain on the medications she'd previously been prescribed, but he added a list of supplements for her to take. He also had several other dietary changes for her to help her with a gluten intolerance issue he'd discovered during her examination.

Rose was skeptical, but she was willing to give it a try. She was told, "Look. What do you have to lose? You've tried everything else. You've only come to see me because I'm your last option. Give the supplements a try. Change your diet. Let's see what happens."

THE THIRTY-DAY TRIAL

Rose promised her husband Tom that she would give it thirty days, and she would hold to her promise. She made the decision then and there that she would try the alternatives, along with the traditional meds for the next month.

Three weeks went by, and she woke up one morning realizing she was feeling better. The improvements had been happening gradually, below the radar. But after three weeks, she could tell her new regimen was making a difference. She made up her mind immediately and there to take her commitment to the next level. She got out of bed and looked at her collection of medications lined up on her nightstand; she picked one of them out and decided not to take it that day. She

A ROSE BY ANY OTHER NAME IS STILL A ROSE: ROSE'S STORY

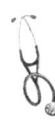

was pleasantly surprised to find that nothing bad happened. Her health continued to improve.

A few days later, she picked out another prescription and eliminated that one from her daily routine. Her improvement continued. With the exception of a few of the pain medications, she was able to wean herself off the traditional medications over the next several weeks. She continued to take the supplements and she kept up with the changes in her diet.

It took nine long months but for the first time in years she found that she was able to go off of the pain medications entirely. It was predicted she'd be in a wheelchair within the year, but with the help of her doctor, she proved all of them wrong. Today Rose knows she'd be in a wheelchair but for the wisdom and treatment she experienced with alternative care.

HITTING CLOSE TO HOME

How does she know? Sadly, Rose has a relative who suffers from some of the very same inflammatory diseases that she has had to deal with in her life. But where Rose wholeheartedly embraced the alternative approach, this relative has clung to the belief that traditional medications alone can help her with her problems.

Rose's relative is ten years younger but is currently confined to a wheelchair and unable to walk without assistance. Rarely does someone get to watch what could have happened if they'd taken another path. With her sister, Rose is continually confronted with what that path could have held in store for her.

The Good Doctor

HIGH HOPES IN OKLAHOMA

Rose's battles were not over. She had other issues to deal with. When Rose was quite a bit younger, she'd had a hysterectomy. Even though this had happened years before, she continued to have to deal with lingering hormonal issues. The doctor told Rose about his colleague and friend...me.

He recommended that she come and see me. But I was still in Coffeyville, and she was in Tulsa. Rose was willing to make the trip if it meant getting some relief from her suffering. Because of his confidence in me, Rose's hope was high. She was confident that I'd be able to help her find some relief.

At the time, I was the only doctor in the area regularly doing hormone treatment. Rose called and made an appointment and eagerly made the ninety-minute trip north to Coffeyville. If her naturopath could use the alternative approach to help her deal with the inflammatory diseases, she was confident I could help her with an alternative approach to her hormonal issues.

By now Rose was familiar with how my colleague practiced medicine, but I'm not sure she was prepared for me. Though he and I were very close, we were also very different in style and bedside manner. Where he was quick to make the prognosis, I tend to be much more thoughtful and deliberate. I ask a lot of questions. In fact, I expect that most people know more about their condition than most doctors. I feel that a good doctor should be a good investigator, asking a lot of questions before arriving at any conclusions.

With Rose, it didn't take long. By first obtaining her history and doing her physical examination, we were able to confirm my hypothesis. With just a few tests we determined that she needed her hormones tuned up. After an injection of a test dose to better define the amount needed, we discussed different applications of hormones and opted for the pellet mode of hormonal replacement. We know the blood levels give us an idea of the dose, but not the sensitivities of the woman's hormone receptors. To decide the correct dose, we give a dose based on their age, size, and symptoms. In this way we are able to closely personalize the dosage to the patient.

Many patients have trouble articulating exactly what's going on in their bodies. I can't count the times I've asked a patient in my office what's wrong with them only to be met with a stuttering response, or worse, a blank stare. My belief is that they've been shut down so many times by doctors practicing traditional medicine they no longer have confidence in their opinion. The patient may go in thinking they know what might be wrong with them only to be shut down by a doctor who makes up his or her mind too quickly. Doctors need to know "his story" or in medical jargon "The History."

In my case, the patient may talk a bit about surface symptoms but in many instances, they are reluctant to give me the whole story. Over the years, I've learned to keep asking and keep probing until the real story begins to emerge. Along with the physical examination, getting the patient's story is a prerequisite for an accurate diagnosis. The taking of a good history has not changed much in the last century. The elements are:

- **Chief Complaint** - what is the main problem that brought the patient to see the physician in the first place?
- **History of Present Illness** - the details of when the illness started, how it started, what brought it on, what

The Good Doctor

is helping, and any related symptoms. (The Symptoms are *how* the patient feels and the Signs are *what* the patient *feels*).

- **Past Medical History** - the previous medical illnesses and surgeries they had.

- **Family History** - health (and death) of parents and siblings can also play a role in genetics, which at times can profoundly influence a person's health.

- **Lifestyle** - occupation, sleep habits, type of food, exercise (or lack thereof), smoking, alcohol intake, soda, fluid intake, habits, etc. are some of the questions a doctor should ask to get the idea of how that person manages their life.

- **The Review of Systems** - a doctor should do a thorough rundown of the list of physio/pathologic issues that an individual may have. These issues could be a direct contributor to the current problem or be a stand-alone issue. There are several ways of doing this, but I start at the top of the head and go down the body to the toes.

    ○ HEAD - aches and pains

    ○ MOUTH - tongue, teeth, throat issues

    ○ EYES - pain, blurry vision, tearing, itching, dryness

    ○ NOSE - sense of smell, running, bleeding

    ○ EARS - acuity, ringing, pain, itching

    ○ SINUSES - congestion, fullness

    ○ NECK - tenderness or pain, swallowing issues

A ROSE BY ANY OTHER NAME IS STILL A ROSE: ROSE'S STORY

- CARDIOVASCULAR - heart area discomfort, irregular or rapid heartbeat, shortness of breath, swelling of ankles, leg muscles hurt when walking, inability to breathe while lying flat, lightheadedness when standing.

- RESPIRATORY - chest pain, shortness of breath (this item figures both here and under heart symptoms), cough, wheeze.

- GASTROINTESTINAL - stomach ache, heartburn, abdominal cramps, good bowel movements, nausea, vomiting, early satiety, hunger pains, dark urine (indicating bile in the urine from liver/gallbladder).

- GENITAL-URINARY - back pains, frequency of urination, burning during urination, getting up more than two times a night to urinate.

- GYN - Gravida (number of live pregnancies), Para (the number of live deliveries), Abortions (the number of times that baby did not go to term). Also how the periods were going - the timing of the cycle, how heavy the flow, how much pelvic pain during or before the menses, change in mood or sleep, etc.

- NEURO-PSYCH - numbness and or burning in extremities, weakness in a particular muscle group, incapability of walking correctly (gait), shakiness, episodes of confusion or inability to think of words, poor memory, sleeping well, depression or feeling blue or helpless, losing the battle of a good life.

- INTEGUMENTERY (SKIN) - rash, bumps or lumps on the skin, discoloration, concerning scars.

The Good Doctor

- MUSCULO-SKELETAL - fatigue, muscle-ache, pains, cramps, loss of volume, deformity of an extremity, swelling/heat and redness of a joint.
- ENDOCRINE - heat or cold intolerance (a symptom of low/high thyroid activity), libido, sexual performance.

Performing a focused medical interview without losing the forest because of all the trees is critical to taking a good medical history. Putting all the bits of information in an understandable format, consistent with the patho-anatomic science of the human body is paramount to making a diagnosis. We do need the minutia of the small parts, but do not want it to blur the larger picture. I feel compelled to *listen actively* rather than *hear passively*. A good physician should be able to, in tandem unilaterally, tense the muscle to the stapedius (an inner ear bone) and relax the muscle to the eardrum on their dominant side, mine being the right ear, to better *listen to the words* of a song. Simultaneously, a good physician should be able to *feel the tune* or the vibrations emanating from the patient's subconscious. Most good doctors I know have this God-given ability to "read between the lines" and make sense out of the patient's clinical portrayal of his or her malady. Asking other pertinent questions to add to the above history will bring about a better diagnosis for the reviewing physician.

FINDING THE HIDDEN CULPRIT

From the time I entered the exam room, my radar was up. I was paying close attention to Rose's demeanor and her gait. I sat on my exam chair and rolled over across the room until we were knee-to-knee. When I shook her hand, I was able to

A ROSE BY ANY OTHER NAME IS STILL A ROSE: ROSE'S STORY

observe how wet her palms were and how loose her finger joints were. Her breath and body odor were all subtle clues to the state of her health even before I asked her the first question of the formal medical interview. I took her hands in mine and began to ask her about her situation.

I believe medical practice is a two-way street, involving both the doctor and the patient. Like I've said, no one knows more about the patient's condition than the patient. I fully expect my patients to be experts when it comes to what's going on with their bodies. I send patients home not only with supplements or medications but usually with a study assignment as well.

With Rose, after only a few moments I deduced that it was her early hysterectomy that was causing her hormonal problems, and I immediately ordered a blood test. Sure enough, the tests came back showing deficiencies in a few specific hormones. I put her on the recommended hormone therapy and Rose experienced immediate relief. To date, Rose has had the hormone pellets inserted in her hip over fifty times and she swears by them.

In April of 2014, Rose contracted lupus. She came back to see me, and I came up with several ideas for her ongoing treatment, none of which sounded right to Rose. She pushed back and sent me to the drawing board more than once. Her interest in her medical plan was incredibly encouraging for me. Rarely do I have a patient willing to work as hard for her healing as Rose was. She encouraged me to come up with something different, something outside the box.

After digging deeper for solutions, I thought of the hormone estriol. Estriol is one of the three main estrogens

The Good Doctor

produced by the human body. It's produced in significant quantities by the placenta during pregnancy. But since Rose had a hysterectomy years ago, she'd never been pregnant, let alone had a baby. It occurred to me that Rose could have an estriol deficiency. This could be the solution we were looking for. But instead of immediately prescribing it, I ran it by Rose. I gave her the assignment to go home and do some studying on her own to see if estriol might be the right solution for her.

After some intense study, Rose was convinced that estriol was just the ticket for her and called me. I immediately set her up to receive treatment by a chiropractor in my clinic, who administers this type of hormone therapy to many of his patients. Rose came into the office and received the IV Estriol therapy. We were thrilled when the symptoms started to disappear. That night she called me to tell me that her pain was gone.

Rose told me that the reason she appreciates coming to me is that she feels like she's in control. She's the one in the driver's seat, not me. I'm there to help and advise, but she's the one in charge. It's not like the more traditional route where the patient is often subjected to whatever the doctors may come up with. Rose says, "With Dr. Block, I feel in control. I know myself and I know when stuff's not right with my body."

I wish all my patients were as engaged and involved in their health as Rose is. Together we were able to come up with a solution that would help her maintain her good health. Rose was thrilled when I decided to move my office from Coffeyville to Tulsa. She continues to come and see me about four times a year, and her drive is a whole lot shorter than it used to be!

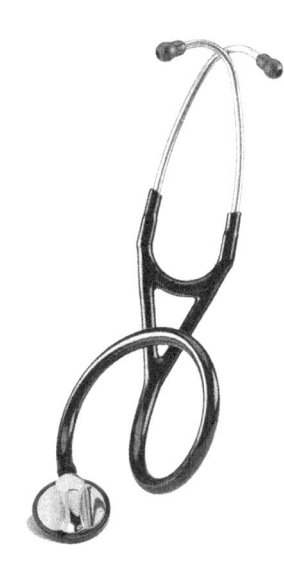

CHAPTER TWELVE:

IS IT WORTH DYING FOR?

It's fairly common to ignore in ourselves the things we focus on so keenly in others. It's like the house painter having the worst looking house on the block or the paint and body man driving a junker. The best of us can fall prey to ignoring the obvious when it comes to ourselves.

This was true with a colleague of mine, Dr. Robert S. Eliot. He founded the Department of Preventive and Stress Medicine at the University of Nebraska Medical Center and later a similar one in Phoenix. This was living proof until he too "died." On a beautiful spring day years ago, this world-renowned cardiologist, then only forty-four, suffered his first heart attack…as he stood on a podium lecturing on "How to Prevent Heart Attacks"!

Here's a stress doctor having a heart attack caused by stress while giving a speech on how to prevent heart attacks! It would be funny if it weren't so sad.

Bob made a full recovery only to die of a fatal event several years later. "If you have a heart attack," he initially joked, "mine

The Good Doctor

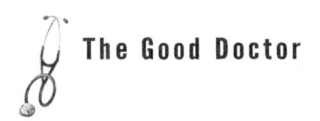

is the kind to have...mild and in a hospital." Over his career, he became one of the major voices of a growing movement to teach people they can be highly productive without allowing stress to destroy their quality of life. Bob was his own first stress patient. Finding his prognosis bleak, he redoubled his efforts to change the players so it would not lead to another episode.

THE STRANGERS WITHIN

Bob discovered the two strangers within himself who were in the continuous throes of a conflict. He began a program of recreation and relaxation and he was no longer "Robert the Robot," as he put it, but a human being who learned to enjoy his family and work as more than props to his own ego.

He did die early in his crusade after becoming a consultant to Fortune 500 firms, foreign governments, and Pentagon officials. Bob led the movement to help folks make stress work for them, not against them. However, other factors were against him, factors that he put on the back burner. These included abnormally high lipids, blood pressure, and homocysteine.

Bob's initial movement has grown and reached the modern world. The management of stress was taken out of psychology, where it has been mired for generations, and put into mainstream medicine, where many feel it belongs.

THE SIGNS OF STRESS

The signs of stress are familiar and troubling: anger, anxiety, and sleeplessness. Along with these come headaches, muscle

IS IT WORTH DYING FOR?

tensions, aches, and poor sleep. But far more severe are the reactions you can't feel. Your body responds to danger, both real and perceived, in ways that have evolved over millions of years and often entirely inappropriate to today's problems. We have many a year in the forest, and just a few on the farm, and even less in the factory. The life we live today, the life of modern technology, has existed for only about the last sixty years.

Depending on the danger, the body responds in one of two major ways. The first is the acute alarm reaction, sometimes known as the fight-or-flight response. If one feels immediately threatened, our body responds by producing chemicals for extra strength and energy. Adrenalin, which races through our body, commands a series of changes: The heart beats faster and stronger and blood pressure rises abruptly, blood is shunted away from the stomach and skin, high-energy fats are rushed into the blood stream, chemicals are released to make blood clot more quickly (in case of injury), the pupils of the eyes dilate, the facial muscles tense, blood vessels in the skin open up, the face flushes, breathing quickens, and blood sugar increases. The body is ready for action.

Primitive man often needed this type of response when he faced a saber-toothed tiger. We sometimes need it too: The fireman charging down the pole, the mother rushing to pull her toddler from oncoming traffic, soldiers in combat, all require an acute alarm reaction. But more often than not, the fight-or-flight response, which can occur anywhere from two to forty times a day, is physiologically inappropriate to such modern-day stresses, such as losing a promotion, losing a lover, or losing anything else important to one's ego.

The long-term vigilance reaction is the body's conservation-withdrawal system. It prepares the body for long-term survival in the face of scarce nutritional resources. It is the body getting ready for cold and storms and days without food, water, and salt. The body is conditioned to conserve vital resources when there is no control over a hostile environment.

When the body is in a state of vigilance, the chemical cortisol moves slowly through and commands a series of changes: Blood pressure rises slowly, body tissues retain vital chemicals such as sodium, high-energy fats are released into the blood, and production of sex hormones is repressed (when you're in danger, you're not thinking of sex). The cortisol increases the flow of gastric acid to aid digestion.

Vigilance sustained too long, however, will weaken the body's immune system against disease. Vigilance can occur on a limited basis if you need to stay up all night to pass your final exams or if you are trying to write a novel while holding down a full-time job. If you are an accountant working night and day during tax season, you will use the vigilance reaction.

But, sadly, vigilance can also be a way of life. The chronically vigilant person may be the air-traffic controller at O'Hare International Airport in Chicago, who has too many planes in the air. Or the person may be a mother who always agonizes over her teenage daughter's whereabouts, sitting up into the wee hours waiting for the phone to ring with the bad news. The person could be anyone who feels that he or she is in a losing situation with no acceptable options to change things, anyone who asks himself that direful question, "Is that all there is?"

Many of us have developed bad psychophysiological habits and go around in a constant state of high stress along with the underlying concern that they will not be successful in life. They have learned to live with high levels of anxiety, including rare panic attacks. They think this condition of psychophysiological arousal is normal. Many present symptoms of irritable bowel, headaches, or high blood pressure. All we can do is to try to "quiet them down" a bit.

LEARNING TO REDUCE STRESS

Biofeedback is a system that makes people aware of how their bodies are reacting to stress. Breathing repatterning can help significantly. While shallow breathing from the chest results in a rapid eighteen breaths a minute, which is a sign of stress and, occasionally, hyperventilation. The deeper breathing from the diaphragm requires only twelve breaths a minute and brings a sense of relaxation and well-being. Electrical activity from the diaphragmatic muscle converts into an audio tone. The patient learns how to recognize when the tone is getting higher, which would be a sign of arousal and stress. They can learn to lower it consciously.

By making the covert overt, biofeedback enables patients to regulate their bodily reactions to stress and, for this reason, gain a sense of reassurance. Some of the patients are astonished to see how their bodies are overreacting to stress. At first some patients who are really uptight and into rigid self-control are frightened by the idea of deep relaxation. Once they learn how to regulate their responses, they think it's great.

Think about it. "Is it really worth dying for?" is the most important question for a stressed-out life and its effects on health and disease. Hot reactors are apparently healthy people who overreact dangerously to such everyday occurrences as losing a tennis game or missing a train. If you are a "hot reactor," you can be responding to stress with an all-out physical effort that takes a heavy toll on your health...without your even being aware of it.

Science has identified that stress is about much more than just emotion. There is now a program for recognizing, reducing, and reversing the hidden effects of stress in our life, to make the stress work for us and not against us!

Scientific evidence has shown that structured therapeutic breathing, if performed without an effort or particular concentration, can significantly lower our blood pressure. However, these effortless therapeutic breathing sessions are difficult to perform on our own without training or continuous, individualized coaching. Learning how to relax is fundamental to self-care. Relaxation with breathing is the antidote for stress caused by the fight-or-flight response. It is the balancing of the involuntary wrestling match between the parasympathetic and the sympathetic nervous system. In our offices, we do a simple EKG/ANSAR study to determine how unbalanced the system is.

RELAX

Real relaxation is a form of concentrated meditation that changes our brain waves from the beta, or thinking state, to the alpha, the relaxed state. If we can get ourselves into this situation for ten to twenty minutes twice a day, we can change virtually every physiological function in our bodies, and, as a result, improve our physical and mental condition. When we temporarily eliminate the mental tug-of-war in our daily routines and allow the body to enter a state of quiet counterpoise, our natural homeostasis, balance, and functional equilibrium begin to prevail. Many techniques are used to foster relaxation. Here are a few simple ones.

Sit comfortably in a quiet room in a chair and uncross your legs and arms to eliminate muscular tension. With your feet on the floor, rest your arms comfortably in your lap or on the arms of the chair. Close your eyes and breathe in through your nose and out through your mouth, allowing your belly to be soft. Try to keep your mind blank; listen to your mind's voice say, "soft" as you breathe in, and "relaxed" as you breathe out. If thoughts intrude, let them come and let them go.

A mantra is the second technique that is used. It comes from Transcendental Meditation, which is of subcontinental Indian origin. A mantra is a particular word we select for ourselves that frequently has a harmonious vibration internally and externally. It is a word that represents harmony with the universe, such as one, peace or love. My personal mantra is "peace." I close my eyes and every time I exhale I see peace, either the word or the letters, p-e-a-c-e, coming out of my mouth like smoke gradually floating up, forming the word.

It's important for the mantra to fit our personal belief systems. Thus, some choose "Jesus," and others, "relax." Although sleep is not part of this process, if time is not a premium, after ten to fifteen minutes many fall asleep and wake up extremely refreshed.

During this period of relaxation, the body rejuvenates continually throughout the day. When a stressful situation arises, I tell my patients to utter their mantra or to go through the action of their mantra for a few seconds. Suddenly, like Pavlov's dogs, a programmed response relaxes the individual.

The Good Doctor

You might remember that Pavlov rang a bell each time he fed a group of dogs. After several days of feeding, he rang the bell, and the dogs would salivate even though there was no food. This is a conditioned response that happens in most animals, including humans. As the highest form of animal, we can learn from the others. Seemingly, dogs know more about self-care than their masters.

Practicing a relaxation exercise, or a mantra, ten to forty-five minutes once or twice a day improves one's outlook, decreases anxiety, lowers blood pressure, and enables the whole body to work better. Plainly, these procedures are useful in the absence of illness, but they can also be applied to many medical diseases. Fertility, for instance, is enhanced, heart disease decreased, and pain syndromes improved, all along with the improvement of our general well-being. If thoughts come, let them go. This removes us from stress and fosters the body's healing. Meditation is also powerful in preventing disease. As a result, it is beginning to come back into the mainstream medical field.

A personal favorite of mine is the HIGH FIVE method. With this method of meditation/relaxation, one inhales through the nose for a count of five, then holds the breath in for a count of five, and then exhales the air through the nose for a count of five. When exhaling, the tip of the tongue should be touching the roof of the mouth, immediately in back of the front teeth. This is the yogic position that most enhances relaxation. I do this procedure five times a day; first thing in the morning, even before getting out of bed. At the end of the day after I say my prayers, plus three times a day when I think about it. If a person does this exercise four times a day they will still be doing well. If it is hard to remember to

IS IT WORTH DYING FOR?

do the exercises, simply do one before each meal. This will also relax you for the forthcoming meal, which will enhance your digestion. This is also a fringe benefit of praying before each meal.

THE MIRACLE OF MUSIC

Listening to certain kinds of music, particularly classical or Gregorian Chants, is also a vehicle for relaxation and healing. For centuries, neuropsychologists have been working to improve the subconscious mind with methods such as neuro-linguistic reprogramming (the unconscious formation of words), and subliminal messaging (speech below the audible threshold).

The melody, pitch, timing, and beat of such music as Pachelbel's "Canon in D," and other Baroque classics along with chants by the Benedictine Monks of Santo Domingo de Silos, can alter your state of being by quieting your mind and allowing you to enter its spiritual recesses.

Most scores of classical music range between 60 and 120 beats per minute. The resting heart beats approximately 50 to 60 times per minute, so it would appear that soothing scores in this range induce calm.

Another type of relaxation with music is "Binaural Beats," the term used for music with slightly different frequencies in each ear. The difference in these frequencies or beats elicits beneficial brain waves by releasing healthy neurotransmitters. So, in addition to drugs (antidepressants, energizers, and sleep aids), binaural music can help stress related or genetically endowed syndromes, such as insufficient sleep, chronic fatigue, fibromyalgia, dyslexia, and ADHD. Improved memory,

The Good Doctor

learning, concentration, and creativity can be heightened by this technique.

By varying the difference of the frequencies in each ear, the brain wave frequency can be ranged from 0 to 100 Hertz, and accordingly affect various parts of the brain. Neurotransmitters such as serotonin (which promotes relaxation and aids eating), noradrenaline (which supports memory and physical performance), dopamine (which affects coordination and addictions), and acetylcholine (which promotes memory with its various expressions) are increased or decreased. If the frequency were 410Hz in the left ear and 400Hz in the other, they would have a ten beat difference, mimicking the Alpha state. But since the rhythm is the same, and there is such a small difference in pitch, the listener just hears the music.

Through the auditory nervous branches and its ramifications, electrochemical energy is transferred to various parts of the brain and entraps their nervous signals. Electroencephalography indicates that both hemispheres become involved with identical frequency with amplitude and coherence. This maximizes the intra-hemispherical neural response so that if one is left-brain dominant (right-handed), this hemisphere communicates with the other for thought processing. If this is performed while asleep, without the chatter of the external environment, the exchange can be enhanced tenfold.

This technique can help us to go from the deepest Delta wave (0 to 4 H), to the moderately deep Theta dream sleep (4 to 8 H), to the twilight Alpha (8 to 14 H), the alert Beta (15 to 50 H) state and the highly focused Gamma state, which is the frequency of an extremely focused athlete or like William Tell, preparing to shoot an arrow at an apple off his son's head. But

IS IT WORTH DYING FOR?

it's in the Delta state that super learning occurs, and the youth giving human growth hormone is released. There are applications for the iPhone for $1.99 that, with ear buds, can inspire you to creativity or mindful meditation and dream-filled sleep. Altered State and AmbiSci are two of the many apps offered.

CDs are also available that are easily inserted into a player with the same effect. (See LifeProgram.com.) For your mental and physical health, consider the music that heals. A device called the RESPeRATE is now available. To deliver effortless therapeutic breathing without any prior training, the RESPeRATE utilizes a patented "Interactive Respiratory Pacing" technology, which ingeniously takes advantage of the body's natural tendency to follow external rhythms.

RELAX WITH RESPeRATE

Using a breathing sensor, RESPeRATE automatically analyzes our individual breathing patterns and creates a personalized melody composed of two distinct inhale and exhale guiding tones, delivered through comfortable earphones.

Just listen to the melody through the headphones and synchronize the breathing to the tones. By prolonging the exhalation tone, RESPeRATE guides the breaths correctly to reach the "therapeutic zone" of less than ten breaths per minute.

The physiological result is the muscles surrounding the small blood vessels in the body dilate, and relax. Blood is allowed to flow more freely, and pressure is directly, significantly lowered. Within three to four weeks of use, a significant, all day reduction in blood pressure can be achieved. And while your breathing returns to normal after each session with

The Good Doctor

RESPeRATE, the beneficial impact on your blood pressure and life is cumulative. With the regular use of the RESPeRATE or a similar design, measurable, sustained reduction in blood pressure could be achieved without medications, and dying earlier in life as detailed by my two colleagues would be avoided.

TARGET: STROKE

Oddly, the most challenging link to shorten is the time between arriving at the ER door and receiving the right treatment. In a large study called "Target Time: Stroke," only 30 percent of patients receiving thrombolytic therapy were treated with a door-to-needle time less than the time recommended by the American Heart Association or the American Stroke Association of sixty minutes.

The findings of Target: Stroke was alarming enough to the medical community to get some much-needed movement. In 2010, an initiative was launched with the goal of decreasing the door-to-needle time. The authors of the study identified ten key strategies to reduce this time and provided hospitals with an implementation manual, support tools, and "best practices" education from other centers. They also provided performance feedback and even opportunities for national recognition. Over one thousand hospitals participated in the initiative with 43,000 patients.

The good news is that by 2013, as a result of the initiative, the median door-to-needle time had dropped from seventy-four minutes to the magic fifty-nine minutes. This reduction in time has not only saved lives, but it has saved the quality of life as well. Another study by the University of Melbourne found that

IS IT WORTH DYING FOR?

each minute saved in the treatment chain provided (on average) an extra 1.8 days of healthy life! That means with each fifteen-minute decrease in treatment delays, it provides the patient with an additional one-month of disability-free life.

These studies are giving us actual numbers to bolster what we all believed to be true in the first place; if you decrease the time until treatment, you increase the chances of recovery. Even small achievements in streamlining stroke services, provide tremendous gains for the patient. When ambulance services, ERs, and stroke teams can work together to decrease these times, lives can be saved.

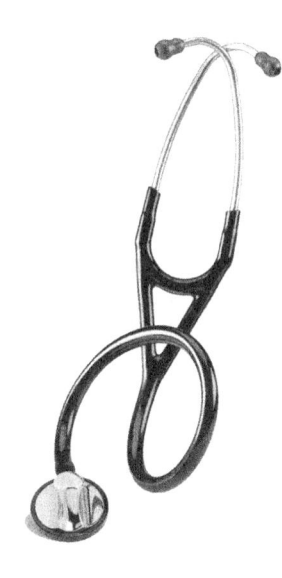

CHAPTER THIRTEEN:
DON'T WORRY! BE HAPPY!

One of the key ingredients to a longer, happier life is an attitude of gratefulness. That's not just my opinion; that's according to research accruing over the last decade. It is good to have an annual holiday, like Thanksgiving or Christmas to remind us to express gratitude, but thankfulness should be an attitude we live with all year round.

People who are thankful for what they have can cope with stress. They have more positive emotions, and they're better able to reach their goals, all of which are associated with improved health and a longer, better life!

ADOPTING THE ATTITUDE OF GRATITUDE

Gratitude is a thankful appreciation for what a person receives. With gratitude, people acknowledge the goodness in their lives. In the process, people usually recognize that the source of all that goodness lies at least partially outside themselves. As a result, gratitude also helps folks connect to something larger than themselves. This connection could be to family, friends, employers, society, or a higher power, as in 1 Chronicles 4:10.

"Jabez cried out to the God of Israel, 'Oh, that you would bless me and enlarge my territory! Let your hand be with me, and keep me from harm so that I will be free from pain.' And God granted his request" (NIV).

As noted above, gratitude could be expressed for things that occurred in the past, but we should also be grateful for the present and future. We retrieve positive memories from our past, and we're appreciative for those past blessings. But we should also be thankful for the gifts of today, as well as tomorrow's expected favors. If we do this, not only hope but also optimism will triumph in our life.

Studies have shown that gratitude can produce a number of measurable effects on our body. These include elevation of mood neurotransmitters (serotonin and norepinephrine), social bonding hormones (oxytocin), cognitive and pleasure-related neurotransmitters (dopamine), and a decrease of inflammatory and immune systems (cytokines) as well as stress hormones (cortisol).

Cultivating a sense of gratitude helps us refocus our attention toward what's good and right in our life, rather than dwelling on the negatives and the things we feel lacking. Starting each day by thinking of all the things for which we have to be thankful puts our mind on the right track. What we think about tomorrow depends to a large extent on what we believe about today. Every moment of every day is an opportunity to turn our thinking around, as we make the conscious choice to think more positively about our future.

Be appreciative for what you have. When life gives you a cause to cry, remember the reasons you have to be happy. Face the past without regret; prepare for the future without fear, but focus on what's good right now—in the present moment. Gratitude is essential to a positive mental outlook.

THE IMPORTANCE OF OPTIMISM

For years, doctors have minimized the importance of a positive mental outlook in a patient's physical health. It's easy for a physician to lose sight of the whole being, becoming so focused on the physical body that he or she loses sight of the emotional factors that can lead to healing. In the same way, a doctor can too quickly relegate happiness to strictly a psychiatric process with no bearing on physical healing. While psychiatrists are indeed trained in the mental and emotional aspects of a person's well-being, it's a critical factor for other doctors to be aware of as well.

It's my belief that happiness brings a life-giving vibrancy to our lives. It's joy that gives us that flow of movement that quickens our pulse and causes us to get out of bed in the morning. It's a positive mental attitude that encourages us to get up and take that first step of the day, and then the one after that and the one after that. I've seen patients with ailments they could easily overcome but because they had lost all hope, which drained their happiness, they gave up, all because they didn't have the right attitude. Likewise, I've seen patients with serious health issues kept alive by their positivity.

The Good Doctor

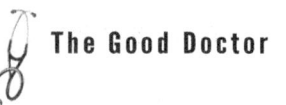

THE DOWNSIDE OF TESTING

In the United States, we are the most over-tested, over-diagnosed and over-treated society in the history of mankind. Brilliant scientists, engineers, and doctors have devised various tests and invented marvelous machines that can detect disease or even the probability of disease long before the illness occurs. While this sounds good on the face of it, often it only serves to foster fear in the mind of the patient. Never forget, fear is the great thief of hope. That's why I maintain that just because we have the ability and technology to do a test, and even have the insurance plan to pay for it, does not mean we should have the test done.

Let me give you an example of what I mean. We've known for some time that when you get a CAT scan, you're exposing yourself to dangerous levels of radiation. Now, researchers have linked almost 200,000 deaths per year to cancers that were caused by the exposure to the radiation emitted during the CAT scans.

There are dangers in other tests as well. The dye used to inject into a patient to get a better look at the blood vessels takes a severe toll on the kidneys. If a patient were to get several of these tests within a short amount of time (more than fifteen tests in less than three years), a 30 percent decline in overall kidney function will occur.

The colonoscopy is another test often given unnecessarily. This test is routinely given every few years once a patient reaches fifty years old. It's not the test I object to as much as the routine nature in which it's given. These tests, in some cases, can perforate the colon, which can cause an infection

DON'T WORRY! BE HAPPY!

within the abdominal cavity. It's staggering to think that one person in seventy will die from complications from these tests.

Yes, you should regularly be tested if your father or uncle had colon cancer. Heredity is a key factor in contracting this type of cancer. But there are tests you can take without the invasiveness of a colonoscopy that will help you determine the odds of you contracting colon cancer. Among these tests is the "Colon Sentry."

If this simple blood test finds that your odds are 1 in 20, then yes, by all means get the colonoscopy. But if your odds were found to be 1 in 1,400, then there's no need to go through the discomfort of this test and expose yourself to the risk of the complications that this test can cause.

Another unnecessary test in my opinion is the PSA, which stands for prostate-specific antigen. Doctors routinely give this test to their male patients as they approach fifty years of age. The PSA is unnecessary as there are other ways to determine the presence of prostate cancer. The only thing the PSA test does is assign a number. The higher the number, the greater the likelihood of cancer. But even the National Cancer Institute says that there is no specific normal or abnormal level of PSA in the blood. Most doctors have assumed that a 4.0 ng/mL or lower is normal. So if the patient were found with a level higher than that, the doctor would be convinced of his need to look for further evidence of prostate cancer. Just like with the colon cancer test, there are better blood studies that would indicate whether to "worry and react" or "wait and relax." Becoming proactive based on a lab report can give a man peace of mind.

In the mid 1980s, Dr's. Ming Chu, Thomas Stamey, and William Catalona established the importance of the PSA in diagnosing prostate cancer. Now fast forward to 2013 when there would be an estimated 238,590 new cases of prostate cancer and 29,720 deaths, making it the second leading cause of cancer death in U.S. men.

Widespread prostate cancer screening using the PSA has led to a dramatic reduction in the proportion of men diagnosed with metastatic disease and prostate cancer death rates. However, PSA screening continues to be highly controversial due to its limited specificity for clinically significant prostate cancer, resulting in unnecessary biopsies for false positive results, as well as detection of some indolent tumors that would not have caused harm during the patient's lifetime.

To preserve the benefits of screening and early detection and to reduce these harms, there has been great progress into alternate ways of using the PSA test with better performance characteristics. These include the unbound form "free PSA," which indicates a greater likelihood that the elevation is from benign conditions rather than prostate cancer. The latest test, which is the proPSA ('p2PSA') is added to the equation.

The Prostate Health Index (PHI) is a new formula that combines all three forms (total PSA, free PSA, and p2PSA) into a single score that can be used to aid in clinical decision-making so the patient can come to an intelligent and informed rather than an ignorant "seat of the pants" conclusion.

In my experience, these "seat of the pants" conclusions do nothing but worry the life out of the poor patient with a slightly elevated number. The language used by their doctor only reinforces the fear stating, "We're going to have to watch this very carefully" or "We'll need to test this every four months now to make sure you don't have cancer." Far more patients will die

DON'T WORRY! BE HAPPY!

with cancer of the prostate rather than *from* cancer of the prostate. The fact is that 90 percent of men who live long enough will develop a few cells of cancer in their bodies before they die.

All of these unnecessary tests and overdiagnoses only serve to decrease the quality of life, which will ultimately shorten the quantity of life. Worry and fear over what might happen or what could occur steals our peace, robs us of hope and happiness, which turns our attitude sour and negative.

Never downplay the importance of the positive mental attitude in the healing process. I would never lie to a patient, but I will strive to be as positive as I can be about their situation.

A DOCTOR'S FIRST BATTLE: FEAR

Often when a patient comes to see me they're scared. Chances are they've already seen other doctors and have been wrestling with their situation for some time. The dark scenarios have been swirling around in their mind causing their stress levels to rise. They're thinking about all the worst-case possibilities. As they begin to explain to me their condition, their radar is up on full alert, searching my face for any telltale clues that will give them the truth about their status.

They're watching my eyes, my eyebrows, and my mouth. They pay close attention to my breathing and posture, looking for any sign that their fear is warranted. I know what it is to struggle with fear. I've been scarred by fear's ugly presence in my life. That's why I pay special care, knowing that my body language, my tone of voice and my inflection are all just as important as the actual words I speak.

The Good Doctor

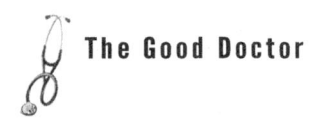

THE FACE OF EMOTION

It's curious, as we consider our facial expressions, how important they are in our communications. But it turns out that our facial expressions control more than just what we communicate; they can drive our emotions as well.

William Shakespeare famously wrote "a face is like a book," and conventional wisdom has it that our faces reveal our deep-seated feelings. But what if the reverse were also right? What if our facial expressions set our moods instead of revealing them? What if there were actual science to support the exhortation, "smile, be happy"?

Like I mentioned in a previous chapter, dermatologic surgeon Eric Finzi has been studying that very question for nearly two decades. In his groundbreaking book (*The Face of Emotion*, 2013) he marshals evidence suggesting that our facial expressions are not secondary to, but rather a central driving force, of our emotions.

Dr. Finzi has identified the six basic emotional expressions as fear, disgust, anger, surprise, happiness, and sadness. These expressions have been shown to be universal in their performance and perception. Recently, a growing number of clinical and functional imaging studies have been aimed at identifying a neural infrastructure for recognizing basic emotion and how facial features impact and shape not only our deeds but also subsequent thoughts and how these thoughts are colored.

For example, when someone following instructions lowers their eyebrows, their mood becomes more negative. If, however, they are advised to raise their eyebrows they become more surprised by their surrounding. If people are instructed to wrinkle their noses, then odors are evaluated as more unpleasant.

Many researchers have confirmed the facial feedback hypothesis. Back in 1872, Charles Darwin and twenty years later, William James proposed the theory of facial expressions feed information back to the brain, influencing our emotions. Voluntary contraction of facial muscles into a smile or a frown can induce feelings of happiness or sadness respectively and affect the emotional appraisal of events. This happens via the autonomic nervous system through the Vagus Nerve, the same nerve that both controls and reflects the heart and gastrointestinal tract.

BOTOX FOR DEPRESSION?

A single Botox injection between the eyes has been found to reduce depression by 50 percent. In the largest randomized double-blind study to date, Dr. Finzi and psychiatrist, Dr. Norman E. Rosenthal, used Botox on depressed men and women. They found that 52 percent of subjects suffering from moderate to severe disease showed significant relief after the injection. These findings help confirm a novel concept for mental health; using facial expressions can influence thoughts and feelings!

The mechanism by which Botox abolishes depression indicates that frowning does affect the way we feel about ourselves when looking in the mirror, but it can even change the way others respond to us. The Botox therapy reduces the level of frowning and causes other people to respond in a way that influences our mood favorably. The happy face stimulates a more positive social interaction. Frowning itself is depressogenic, and the reduction therefore is therapeutic.

The Good Doctor

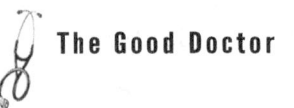

Science knows that the brain continuously monitors the relative ups and downs of facial expressions and that mood responds accordingly. Finzi and Rosenthal term this emotional proprioception. Proprioception is the senses of position and movement of our skin, muscle, tendons, limbs, and trunk. It gives the detection of effort, identifies force, and recognizes gravity. Proprioception uses receptors located throughout our body to feel our internal bodies as they relate to the outside.

This represents an important window to see into our brain's emotional state. Accordingly, the brain continuously assesses the extent of facial muscle contraction and muscle tension by proprioception. The state of our facial muscle tension is part of a neuronal circuit involving the brainstem, with the motor input from the facial nerve and sensory input from facial and trigeminal cranial nerves.

All of this is monitored by the wandering Vagus Nerve that lets our guts and heart know what is going on. That way the inside better knows what is happening on the outside. Botox interrupts the normal circuitry, reduces distress signals to the brain, and by that influences the mood favorably. For this reason "defrowning" modifies our emotional perception and response.

After reviewing the literature, we are starting to offer Botox in our offices, not for cosmetic reasons, but for the treatment of depression. We're using Botox alone or in conjunction with anti-depressive medications as a three-pronged attack that includes psychotherapy as well. We are committed to helping people improve their attitudes and their lives. It's much easier to stay well if you are happy and stress-free!

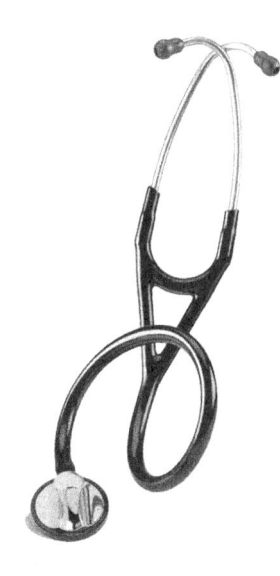

CHAPTER FOURTEEN:
MARRIED TO MEDICINE

Ever since I can remember, the practice of medicine has been my one true goal. I have worked hard to earn the money and even harder to earn the grades to make it into medical school. With my years at the New Jersey College of Medicine drawing to a close, it was time for me to choose an internship.

I had done well throughout my years in medical school and because of that I knew I would have several options on where to do my internship. More than anything else, I felt it was time to get out of the northeast. I was born there, had grown up and gone to school there. I wanted a change. I applied to eleven different general internships, ten of which were in California and the other was in Texas.

I had always been enthralled by the idea of the horse and buggy doctor. I still am to this day. I know it's a romanticized view of medicine, but I wanted to be like one of those brave souls of yesteryear who didn't turn every difficult case over to a specialist. These doctors practiced by instinct, whether it was delivering babies or helping to pass kidney stones. They treated everything from a ruptured appendix to skin rashes and everything in between. That's what I wanted to do! The science and practice of medicine was so fascinating to me I could hardly limit myself to just one part of the body. I wanted to be involved in everything—the whole process! That's why, out of all the directions I could've gone, I chose Internal Medicine as my specialty.

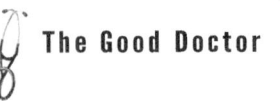

Internal Medicine deals primarily with the prevention, diagnosis, and treatment of adult diseases. These Internal Medicine physicians are especially skilled in the management of patients who have undifferentiated or multi-system diseases. This term *internal medicine* comes from the German term *"Innere Medizin,"* popularized in Germany in the late 19th century to describe physicians who combined the science of the laboratory with the mind, body, and spirit in the care of patients.

Many early 20th century American doctors studied medicine in Germany and brought these complimentary treatments to the United States. Thus, the name "internal medicine" was adopted in imitation of the existing German term. Internists are qualified physicians with postgraduate training in internal medicine and should not be confused with "interns," who are doctors in their first year of residency training.

Although internists may act as primary care physicians, they are not "family physicians," "family practitioners," or "general practitioners," whose training has not solely been on adults. These may include surgeons, obstetricians, and pediatricians.

Although the American College of Physicians defines internists as "physicians who specialize in the prevention, detection, and treatment of illnesses in only adults," I do treat some children who are difficult to diagnose, or children with diagnoses that are resistant to mainstream medicine.

I had been accepted to all eleven internship programs to which I'd applied. When it came time for me to choose which program to attend, the inspiration came from an unlikely place, primetime television.

THE PULL OF BEN CASEY

I never had time to watch much television, but one show I would always try to view was Ben Casey. The show was a medical drama series that ran on ABC from 1961-1966. The show was set in a large Los Angeles hospital. The characters and the plot lines were riveting to me. I could see myself living and working in a large hospital in L.A.

So, it's no surprise that the program I chose was at L.A. County General Hospital, which, at the time, was the largest hospital in the world with over 5,000 beds. The hospital was affiliated with not just one but two medical schools, University of Southern California and Loma Linda University.

The internship program was enormous. It had eight Internal Medicine internships available while at the same time offering over two hundred General Medical internships. It was an honor for me to be chosen for one of the eight Internal Medicine internships.

Internship in medical training is no longer in vogue. That first year after medical school is referred to as a Residency or PGY 1 (Post Graduate Year 1), etc. After this there is another three to five years of training needed, especially in special-

The Good Doctor

ized areas like cardiology. These subspecialties are called fellowships. A young doctor may spend an additional three to five years in perfecting their studies in that specific academic. This is not to be confused with becoming a "Fellow" in that specialty.

Becoming a Fellow is an honor bestowed upon physicians who not only do the academic work and pass their specialty boards but they also are elected by a group of their peers called a "College." This is a legal appointment, and they can use that designation after their MD or DO.

I have a FACP after my MD, which stands for Fellow of the American College of Physicians. If I were a surgeon my FACS designation would be Fellow of the American College of Surgeons, and so on. There are at least sixteen other specialties. A ceremony complete with a gown and cap is a part of the annual meeting of that group.

When I was finally able to start my internship and put the designation of "MD" in my signature, I felt I had arrived. I was busy every day doing the thing I loved most in the entire world. But it wasn't easy. I was only paid $235 per month. The problem was that my rent was $200 a month. That didn't leave much for other needs like utilities, gas, and groceries. I knew I was going to have to moonlight in order to make ends meet. I was no stranger to working hard. But now instead of selling ice cream or encyclopedias I was able to do work I loved for other doctors in my spare time.

I worked doing patient histories and physicals for other physicians. As I think back on those days, it seems all I did was work and study, study and work. I would put in thirty-six hours straight and only get twenty-four hours off to recover. It was hard work, but I loved every minute.

MARRIED TO MEDICINE

After the first year of internship, I was given the license to practice medicine. I went into general practice with Dr. Harold Friese, who was much older than I. Even though I was still working full time in my training program, I received my California medical license and was allowed to have a private practice. I worked as a general practitioner and maintained an office and, because many of my patients were very ill, I had a position in the local community hospital, Garfield Hospital in Monterey Park, California.

Not only would I make as many as fifteen house calls in a day, I would also practice my area of expertise in the hospital, where I was also exposed to a full menu of other issues like heart attacks, hemorrhage, and pneumonias. I was also assisting in surgeries and delivering babies.

The last baby I ever delivered was only one year after I started practice. It was a first-time mother who had been in labor for over thirty-six hours. Although I had delivered over two hundred babies and was trained in applying forceps, I could not bring this one out no matter what I tried. The problem was a persistent "occiput anterior," meaning that the baby's head did not naturally "unscrew" as it descended the birth canal. The poor infant was literally stuck en route to his life. This was a small general hospital outside of a major city and there were no obstetricians on staff. I was the only hope for that baby and mother! Although the baby did make it out alive, it was limp and blue at birth with an APGAR score of only 2.

Virginia Apgar, an anesthesiologist, invented the Apgar score in 1952 as a simple method to quickly summarize the health of a newborn immediately after birth. The Apgar scale is determined by evaluating the newborn baby on five simple criteria, which are, Appearance, Pulse, Grimace, Activity, and

The Good Doctor

Respiration. From each of these the infant is given a score of 0, 1, or 2. The scores are added up and the total sum is their Apgar score. The score is taken routinely sixty seconds and then again five minutes after the birth.

In this case, the baby who was limp and blue at birth was not breathing, nor did it appear to have a heartbeat. In that moment, I felt my heart had stopped beating as well. I resuscitated the baby just like I was taught in my training. Fortunately, I was successful. As you could imagine I carefully followed that child as a patient over the next four years until I changed my venue. The child never had a functional deficit and I was indeed relieved.

But I know now that if I had previously delivered 2,350 babies instead of only 235 babies, I would have had the experience required to successfully rotate that baby myself, speeding up that delivery and lessening the risk to both mother and child.

So from that day forward, I promised myself that I would be as well trained and prepared as possible to take care of the people who put their lives in my hands.

At the time, I was making about $80,000 a year, a pretty good living in those days. I was totally immersed in medicine. In addition to my full-time internship program, I was moonlighting at another private hospital ER. I would work in yet another private hospital all day on Saturdays and Sundays, and then make house calls in the evening when I'd get off work. Yes, I would grab my little black bag and make ten to twelve house calls a night. There was just one problem...

It was against university residency policy for me to moonlight this way.

SWIMMING UPSTREAM

I'll have to admit, it makes sense. If you're still learning to be a doctor, you shouldn't be able to moonlight as a physician! But I was never one to follow the rules too strictly. I always seemed to be the guy who was willing to do whatever it took to see more and do more, even if it didn't follow the letter of the law.

I was totally consumed by my passion. I would finally get home at night, eat a leftover dinner, and briefly connect with my wife before falling into bed about midnight. I learned to repeat my college study habits by waking up at 2:00 and reading between 2:00 and 4:30 when the house was quiet. Then I'd go back to bed until 5:30 when I'd get up and go to work. I would also read on the weekends if I wasn't working. My appetite for more medical knowledge was insatiable.

Although I was learning and growing as a physician and I was making a good living, my superiors had become aware of what I was doing and sat me down for a talk. I was excelling and loving every minute and had even been voted as the Resident of the Year, but my superiors told me they wanted me to stop moonlighting so I could focus more on my residency, which was probably a good idea. Not only was my moonlighting practice against university policy, but it was also ruining my family life. I was indeed married to medicine. As I look back on those years, I regret spending so little time with my family. At the time, I was so full of myself. I thought I was bulletproof, and even though I was pressured by my superiors and my wife to stop the moonlighting, I dismissed their warnings and continued to do as I pleased.

The Good Doctor

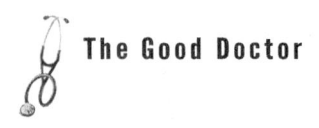

MY UGLY PRIDE

As my pride and arrogance grew, they began to cause real problems. I was spending all my free time devouring medical journals like the Journal of the American Medical Association (JAMA). I'd meticulously go through each journal and read the articles that caught my attention, ripping out and saving many, filing them away for more study later. This was a practice I learned from one of my mentors, Dr. Harold J. Jeghers, who was responsible for getting me the internship at L.A. County General Hospital in the first place. It was Dr. Jeghers who taught me the importance of staying on the cutting edge of current research. Dr. Jeghers had firmly adopted the custom of cutting articles from medical journals and stapling them together. What motivated this activity was the opportunity to utilize the collection of articles in improving clinical teaching, which demonstrates the well-known Samuel Johnson proverb, "Knowledge is of two kinds: we know a subject ourselves, or we know where we can find information upon it."

Dr. Jeghers believed that a physician improved the quality of medicine through self-directed medical education and life-long learning. He held this tenet decades before state medical licensing required continuing medical education. It was Dr. Jeghers who said, "The brain is a thinking organ, not a memory organ, and an effective physician must know how to seek out critical information to solve problems from the voluminous and complex medical literature." I was only just recently able to bring myself to throw away the articles I've clipped over the last fifty years. In the age of the Internet, clipping and filing all those articles has become obsolete!

MARRIED TO MEDICINE

In those days I would study a disease backwards and forwards, not only from traditional textbooks but a historical perspective as well. I would study Harrison's History of Medicine, which was our "bible" of disease diagnosis and treatment. I would go back to the ripped out pages in my files and pour over any of the latest articles on the topic. By the time I showed up for rounds I was overflowing with the most recent knowledge on a variety of diseases and other medical ailments.

It wasn't long before I began to engender hostility with "attending physicians." An attending physician is a well-respected specialist in their field with vast knowledge and experience. In many cases, an attending physician has written significant medical articles and even penned textbooks in their area of expertise. But as these doctors grew older, it seemed to me that many did not have the time and energy to keep up with the latest research.

When I was the senior resident, my group of medical house staff (medical students, interns, junior residents) would do our rounds under the supervision of our attending physician. He would do his best to teach us the details and nuances of each case. We would all study the patient history and come up with our own ideas about the best course of action moving forward.

Because of all the reading I was doing, it wasn't odd at all for me to have several more novel ideas of ongoing treatment than the other house staff, or even the attending physician. I would dive into my files, pulling out articles like ammunition and "showing up" my supervisor, suggesting alternative courses of action. In my arrogance, I would even challenge my supervisor following rounds by asking, "Why didn't you suggest doing this latest diagnostic test?" as I pulled out an article I'd read. Or, "Why did you treat the patient with this

The Good Doctor

already FDA-approved drug for 'off label' use in this diagnosis?" Or, "In yesterday's JAMA there was an article that detailed the true mechanism of the disease we've just seen in this patient!"

I became impatient with their pie in the sky platitudes, their old routines, and traditional ways. I wanted to do new things, explore new ideas, and discover better ways of taking care of the specific patients I was seeing. Sadly, I had become a thorn in the side of my superiors. They were our teachers and they were in charge of grading their house staff, who are the young MDs paid for by the hospital. They're the ones who carried the burden of actually caring for patients while they were learning. By the end of my second year, when contracts for the final year are offered to residents, they'd had enough of my act.

It was like flunking fifth grade all over again! They "canned me," and that word spread to those I worked most closely with; the junior residents, interns, and medical students whom I had taught and made friends with over the three previous years. I was shocked and humiliated. I didn't know if I was going to be able to find another position that would allow me to complete my life's desire. In order to become the best doctor I could, I needed to find an excellent medical facility with a world-class faculty.

I was told to go see the chief of medicine, Dr. Charles Brem. I was ushered into his dark paneled, richly appointed office and asked to take a seat. I sat down in the leather side chair and tried my best to appear at ease. He barely acknowledged my presence. He was engrossed in the papers on his desk, which happened to be my file. Finally, he looked up and took off his reading glasses.

He cleared his throat and looked me dead in the eye. This was not a happy man. My behavior had caused waves in the department and the complaints had worked their way up the chain of command to the very top. I had managed to make the wrong guy very unhappy.

He said, "I make no bones about it, Dr. Block. You're probably a very good doctor. You obviously know your stuff. But the fact is, we don't want you here. You've proven not to care much about the way we do things. You flaunt the fact that you moonlight and make money on the side even though you know it's against university policy. You continually show up your attending physician and undermine his authority in front of the other residents by telling them he doesn't know as much as he should. It's for these reasons that I've decided to end your residency here. You are hereby released from our program."

I was stunned! Didn't he know who I was? I had been voted Teaching Resident of the Year by my medical students! I knew more than our attending physician and I was the one being canned! I was too immature at the time to realize that my pride was the problem. My massive ego had gotten in the way of my becoming an excellent doctor.

THE GIFT I STILL TREASURE TO THIS DAY

The news hit me like a ton of bricks. It was almost the worst day of my life. I thought flunking that history test in college was bad. This was infinitely worse! There was so much more at stake now. I was crushed. But before I left the program, Dr. Paul Worley, who was one of my attendings and knew me well, as chief of both Pediatrics and infectious diseases, gave

The Good Doctor

me a gift I'll treasure forever. He knew about my dismissal and asked me to come see him.

He sat me down and said, "Jerry, what you did wrong was to tell people what they didn't want to hear. The things you said weren't necessarily wrong. It was the way you said them that was in error. You weren't lying. But it was the attitude in which you shared them that people had such a problem with. You know what happened? You let your ego get in the way. You were talking down to doctors who have many more years of experience than you do and you never took any of that into account. You have to learn to control your ego and pride or you'll be out of medicine for good."

He then reached into his top desk drawer and pulled out a small paperback book that would end up changing my life. I had read massive medical textbooks and detailed medical journals, hundreds of them. But nothing changed my life like this little book, *How to Win Friends and Influence People* by Dale Carnegie. He told me, "Don't just read this book, Jerry. Memorize it!"

In less than three hundred pages, Carnegie taught me how I'd used my knowledge, not for good, but to drive people away. By trying hard to prove I knew more, I had caused people to shut down and block me out. My pride had inhibited whatever ability or insights I might have had and kept me, or my ideas, from being considered. I had exercised very little consideration for others, and now they were returning the favor.

Carnegie's book, which I still treasure to this day, taught me a lot about human relations...how people relate to one another. The book taught me how to walk humbly, deferring to others. I am eternally grateful to Dr. Worley for the gift of that book. It saved my career.

A BRAND-NEW START

I needed to begin the process of rebuilding my reputation, but I had to look for another residency program to get into first. I had burned all my bridges at L.A. General. The medical community is a relatively tight-knit one, and word about me had gotten around. There weren't many medical programs interested in stepping up to give another chance to a brash know-it-all.

Fortunately, the program at UCLA, affiliated with Harbor General Hospital, took a chance and accepted me. One of their residents had to drop out because of an illness, leaving an open spot. I would be allowed to take that place, under one condition. I would be on probation and under their microscope every minute of the day. I was going to have to prove that I had indeed turned over a new leaf. I would have to show them that I was no longer the same resident who caused such problems at L.A. General. I had made some significant changes. I was different now and couldn't wait to prove it.

I changed my attitude, and that changed the way I related to others. I no longer tried to show off all I knew. I went out of my way to affirm others and I only offered alternative approaches when I was asked my opinion. I humbly corrected others only when necessary, and I no longer threw the mistakes of others back in their faces.

Not surprisingly, the new approach worked! Together with more hard work and insights I'd learned from Carnegie's book,

The Good Doctor

I was able to prove to my colleagues and my superiors that I had changed. I rose through the ranks once again and was voted the Resident of the Year at Harbor General in 1967. They even asked me to stay for another year and help supervise and train others.

Harbor General was no small program. It was the second teaching hospital for UCLA and at the time, had more applicants for interns and residents and saw more patients than anywhere else in the country.

The position at Harbor also included a teaching assignment at UCLA. I received great training at Harbor General and had the opportunity to expand my teaching experience at a great university. In addition to my teaching, I was appointed Assisting Chief of Emergency Medicine at Harbor General. I was now in charge of overseeing the entire department including about three hundred employees and nurses. I would see a full load of patients as well as supervising the residents.

By God's grace, I was a success. I was made Teacher of the Year in 1968. This repaired some of my bruised ego from sixteen months previous. To me, the award was an acknowledgement of the dozen years I had spent since high school working hard learning and finally succeeding in becoming a good doctor, my trade of choice. I valued this award almost as much as I cherished receiving my MD degree four years earlier. I was able to rub shoulders and even unintentionally compete with other well-respected doctor-teacher-professors who taught with me. I was learning from the best. Some of these other doctors had been considered for the Nobel Prize in medicine earlier in their careers!

MARRIED TO MEDICINE

I had learned my lesson and no longer tried to get ahead by stepping on or over others. I had also given up moonlighting in private practice. I had made up my mind I was going to toe the line. I was making a good living, not as good as in my moonlighting days, but at least I was following the rules. It was well worth it for the peace of mind it gave me.

I loved being a teacher, but I didn't put in all that hard work or travel all those miles just to be a teacher. I wanted to be a doctor! If it was the image of Ben Casey that drove me to California, it was the image of the horse and buggy country doctor that caused me to look eastward to the Midwest for the next chapter of my medical career.

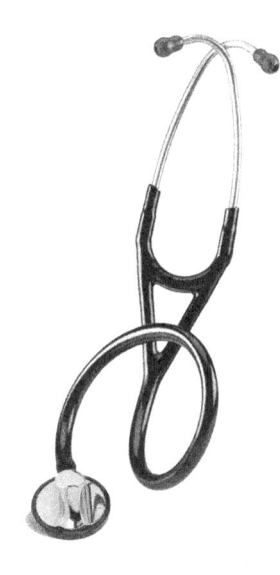

CHAPTER FIFTEEN:

ON TO MISSOURI

I'm a staunch believer in effective goal setting and working hard to achieve the goals you set for yourself. I believe most of us fall short only because we're not willing to work hard enough to see those things we desire in life to come to pass. In my mind, it's often not about ability or talent or skill. It's about focus and hard work.

I've talked a lot about the single-mindedness it took in order for me to become a doctor. My focus and stamina allowed me to work harder than I've ever worked in my life to be the best doctor I could be. At times it seemed that I put in more hours at the office, in the hospital, and my home office studying medicine, than there were hours in the day. But I had a goal in mind and I was able to put all my energies into accomplishing that objective.

But achieving the goal did not come without a lot of sacrifices along the way. There are only so many hours in a day and you only get out of something what you're willing to put in.

The Good Doctor

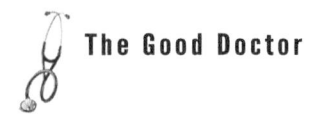

Sadly, because I was unwilling to put much time or energy for my family, they suffered greatly.

Like I said before I was, in many ways, married to medicine. The practice of medicine is the one true passion of my life. For over fifty years, it has been this quest that has gotten me up in the morning to go to work...or up in the middle of the night to study or care for a dying patient. It's where I've spent practically all my time and my energies. I've gotten an enormous amount of fulfillment and satisfaction from the practice over the years.

The fact is, I simply didn't give the time or energy to my first marriage that I should have. It was becoming evident that my wife was not happy. I was never home and even when I was home I was totally consumed by my studies. There simply weren't enough hours in the day for me to go to school, earn a living, and be a proper husband and father to my family.

It was during these times that I first became aware of the hairline cracks that were developing in the foundation of our family. It was a very difficult time. It was time for a new start. We needed a new beginning in a brand-new place. I was sure that once I was in a practice of my own, my time would even out and I'd be able to shore up the cracks in my marriage. I was confident everything would be okay once we got away from the hustle and bustle of life in California.

FOLLOWING ROWDY

Just like Ben Casey attracted me to California, it was another popular television show of the day that directed my attention eastward. The program was Rawhide, starring a very

ON TO MISSOURI

young Clint Eastwood as Rowdy Yates. The show centered on a team of cowboys or "drovers" driving cattle along the Sedalia Trail from San Antonio, Texas, to Sedalia, Missouri. The version of Sedalia portrayed on television looked like the perfect spot for a country doctor.

I made the decision. I told my wife that's what I wanted to do. Soon we were, "On to Missouri!"

It was much easier for me to see myself as a horse and buggy doctor in a place like Sedalia, Missouri, than it was in Los Angeles, California. I began to look for an opportunity to set up shop in Sedalia. I answered an ad posted from a doctor looking for a partner in his practice. When I contacted him, he told me, "Son, if you work real hard you should be able to see about twenty patients a day!"

I knew immediately we weren't on the same page. At the time, I was routinely seeing twenty-five to thirty patients a day in California. I knew then that our pace of work wouldn't match up. So I countered his offer of employment with an offer of my own. I said, "Instead of me coming to work for you, how about if you rent me space in your office and I establish a practice of my own?" That way I would have the independence to be able to work at whatever pace I wanted. He agreed to the deal, and we started the process of moving our family across the country.

Moving to Missouri from Southern California was quite a culture shock to my young family. At the time, the city of Los Angeles population was over 2.5 million people. And that's just the city of Los Angeles proper, not the entire metropolitan area. By sharp contrast, the population of Pettis County, Missouri, of which Sedalia is the county seat, wasn't even 25,000 back then. Yes, it was a culture shock indeed.

The Good Doctor

I expected the slower pace to be a healing balm to my marriage, but only because I had assumed that my pace would match the slower pace of Sedalia. But I continued to run at a high rate of speed and my practice responded to the hard work. By the end of that first year, I saw way too many patients and my practice quickly outgrew the space I was renting from the other doctor. I was forced to expand and build a new, larger office to handle the growth.

The growth was good and I took it as a sign of success. But it wasn't just my office that was monopolizing my time. I was the only Board-certified Internist for the surrounding population of over 100,000. Doctors in towns and cities from miles around were sending me their patients because of my expertise and certification.

Because of my intense interest in Cardiology, I opened the very first coronary care unit in the area. I was also Chief of Medicine for the hospital's ICU. I would supervise, read, and advise on all EKG's done in that hospital. I would also read and advise on the results of all the hospital's stress tests. I would see twenty to thirty patients in the hospital, not only the heart patients but the sick ones from the ICU as well. Then I would see my normal load of thirty patients a day in my practice in my office. I did this day after day, week after week, year after year. The crushing weight of busyness had followed me east to Missouri.

I FAILED MY MARRIAGE

My problem was, I couldn't turn it off. I had an insatiable curiosity and was always on a quest for more knowledge. Often

ON TO MISSOURI

I wouldn't get home until long after my family had gone to bed, 11:00 or later. I would be grouchy, grumpy, and mean-spirited. I'd go straight to bed. But then, as was my long-held habit, I would drag myself out of bed at 1:00 or 2:00 and study for an hour or two before going back to bed for a few hours. But what little sleep I got was often interrupted, because I was the head of the ICU I often got calls at home. I was caught up in a violent whirlpool and didn't know how to free myself.

It wasn't long before the cracks in my marriage became deep with profound fault lines. My wife had had enough and looking back; I can hardly blame her. My marriage was over. She made the decision to leave and take our younger children with her. My oldest daughter was already enrolled at Stephens College, which is a women's college in Columbia, Missouri, so she would remain close while the rest of my family moved away.

I was withering on the vine. My practice, the very thing I loved, was now turning on me. I was never going to last working at this rate. My marriage had now failed and if I continued the way I was going, I was going to kill myself with work. I had to get some help.

I hired another doctor to work in my office and help handle some of the load. But this didn't end up being the solution I was hoping it would be. Not only was the other doctor my backup, I was his. So when he would take time off or get sick, I would have to fill in for him. I would have to see all his patients, in addition to my own. I was still working way too much.

As you can imagine, my daily routine during that time was pretty crazy. Making the rounds at the hospital, reviewing patient records and test results, then going to my office and

The Good Doctor

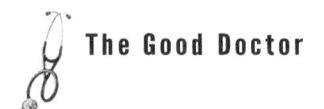

seeing patients there would fill virtually every moment of every day.

A FRESH VOICE FOR A FRESH START

A fact of life for every practicing doctor is the never-ending stream of pharmaceutical sales people traipsing through their doors to make sales calls. They drop by the office at the most inopportune times and want to talk and leave a few samples. With a pretty extensive sales background of my own, I knew how important it was to get in to see the decision-maker. But I had no time to see all the sales people who wanted to tug at my limited time. I had little patience for those who would try to wriggle their way past my team to get into my office. Sales people would be stopped at the front desk and told to leave their literature there. I would research the literature later without the interruption and keep up with all the latest medications and procedures on my own time.

One day I was making the rounds through the hospital and I heard the most beautiful voice. What caught my ear initially wasn't the words that were being spoken, it was the way they were spoken...it was the accent. I grew up in Atlantic City surrounded by Jewish Europeans who were fleeing Hitler's rampage. The German accent was a soothing and familiar sound to me because of all the Germans who had settled in the Atlantic City area during those difficult years.

I followed the voice down the hallway and into an office. It turned out that the voice belonged to a pharmaceutical representative who had brought donuts to the hospital to "bribe" the doctors. She was drop-dead gorgeous and I was immediately

ON TO MISSOURI

smitten, not only with her lovely Bavarian accent but with her beauty as well! Over the next few weeks, I began to see her quite a bit. She was able to do what my first wife couldn't do. She was able to get me to think of something other than my medical practice. I spent as much time with her as I could. I learned that I could step away from the many medical chores I had saddled myself with and still be okay. I never knew there was such life outside the hospital or doctor's office door. Being with her was pure bliss.

We were married six months later.

We're still married today, and it's still the same; every day is pure bliss.

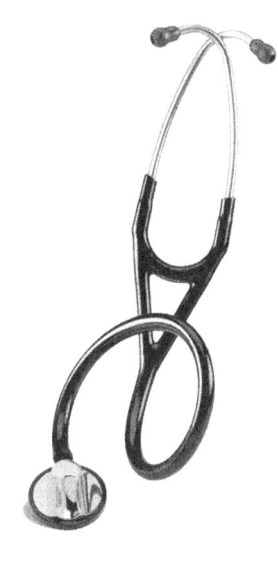

CHAPTER SIXTEEN:

THE NODES HAVE IT: THE JOHN CASTRO STORY

Over the course of my career, I've had the good fortune to find myself in just the right place at just the right time to help someone desperately in need. John Castro's story is one such occasion.

I first met John through his wife Dawn, who was a patient of mine. We ran into each other while having a meal in a local restaurant where Dawn worked. I had no idea that the next time I saw John that his life would be hanging in the balance.

It was February 13, 2013, the day before Valentine's Day. The day was frigid and John felt every bit of that chill. He was cold all day long and no matter what he tried, he couldn't seem to get warm. The chill went all the way to his bones. He was so

The Good Doctor

cold that he decided he probably needed a new, much warmer coat. He went out and bought a brand-new heavy Carhartt coat.

But even the heavier coat didn't cut the chill. When he got home from work, he went straight to bed but woke up in the middle of the night shivering. He knew he must have a fever and thought he was probably struggling with the early stages of a severe cold or the flu, which had been going around at the time.

Over the next few days, John stayed in bed, taking over-the-counter flu medications and hoping to simply sleep it off. But whenever he would try to get out of bed, he'd lose his balance and fall over. John knew that something wasn't right, but he still thought it was simply a case of the flu and that if he'd continue to rest and take his medications, he'd get better. Three long days passed and John wasn't seeing any improvement at all. Dawn was concerned and, not knowing what else to do, made an appointment with my office for an exam and some blood tests.

Both John and Dawn came in for the office visit. I greeted John, recognizing him from our previous meeting in the restaurant. I could tell by looking at him that he wasn't doing well. He was weak and having trouble with his balance. In addition, the constant fever was taking a toll on his body.

FINDING THE CLUE: OSLER'S NODES

When I shook John's hands, I noticed purplish nodules on the pads of his fingers and after several minutes of conversation with him about his condition, I was certain I knew what was wrong with him. I recognized the purplish nodules as

THE NODES HAVE IT: THE JOHN CASTRO STORY

Osler's nodes, of which I'd read about fifty-five years before, but until that day had never seen. These nodules are characteristic of bacterial endocarditis, a fatal disease unless diagnosed and treated immediately.

To hospitalize a patient whose condition didn't look nearly as serious as it was can be tough and take quite a bit of explaining. I copied all my notes down about Osler's nodes for John to give to the doctor at the hospital. I described how Osler's nodes are mysterious signs, spread by the blood to various parts of the body including the finger pads. I recommended blood cultures be taken and that John be given antibiotics immediately.

"Osler's Nodes" is just one example of eponyms that doctors use as a convenient way to label a disease, symptom, or syndrome. Eponyms have become a long-standing tradition in Western science and medicine and being awarded an eponym is regarded as an honor. Doctors often use the quote, "Eponymity, not anonymity, is the standard!"

That's why symptoms, physical findings, diseases, syndromes, and laboratory tests are often referred to by the name of the discoverer of that particular malady, usually publishing their findings in a medical journal. In rare cases, an eponymous disease might be named after a patient. Probably the most famous example would be "Lou Gehrig's Disease" or "Hartnup Disease." William Osler was among the most famous doctors of his time with his name being associated with over thirty diseases, symptoms, or syndromes.

William Osler, who practiced medicine in the late 1800s and the first two decades of the 1900s, is not only famous for his eponyms, he has some great quotes to his credit, a few of which are:

The Good Doctor

- "Medicine is learned by the bedside and not in the classroom. Let not your conception of disease come from words heard in the lecture room or read from the book. See, and then reason and compare and control. But see first."

- "The good physician treats the disease; the great physician treats the patient who has the disease."

- "The practice of medicine is an art, not a trade; a calling, not a business; a calling in which your heart will be exercised equally with your head. Often the best part of your work will have nothing to do with potions and powders, but with the exercise of an influence of the strong upon the weak, of the righteous upon the wicked, of the wise upon the foolish."

- "We are here to add what we can to life, not to get what we can from life."

- "To study the phenomenon of disease without books is to sail an uncharted sea, while to study books without patients is not to go to sea at all."

I COUGH NO MORE

Sometimes a good doctor has to be a good doctor to himself. After two months of a continued minimally or nonproductive cough, I had enough! I did the usual to include hydration, cough lozenges, humidifier, two rounds of antibiotics, a short course of steroids, and a medical evaluation that included a chest X-ray and blood work. Still there was no relief and no other obvious cause. Surely, there had to be a better modality to handle this frustration.

THE NODES HAVE IT: THE JOHN CASTRO STORY

I am writing this to share my newfound knowledge of a "cure" for my nonspecific cough. Like most of these situations, a virus that inflamed my bronchial-tracheal tree initiated the cough. As the infection started to heal, it caused minimal local irritation. This is similar to a small skin lesion such as a pimple. On that surface, the nervous system interprets the stimulus as an itch, which we would intentionally scratch. But in my respiratory structures, it caused a "tickle" that demanded removal. Unable to physically rub or scrap it with fingers, humans do this naturally with a cough.

Perhaps the first little cough spells some relief, but like the skin, it irritates as well giving further inflammation of the area and again causes more of that annoyance. The more a skin lesion is scratched, the better it feels—until a point where it starts to burn, then hurt, and the tissue starts to break down. The physiology is that the more the receptors discharge, the lower their threshold is for the cough/tickle response and the easier they are to cause the same irritating reflex. After a period of time, this degenerates to a vicious downhill course and may never get lasting relief.

A cough, which is reflexive or voluntary, is a sudden and frequently repetitively occurring event. This serves to clear the large breathing passages from secretions, irritants, foreign particles, and microbes. The cough reflex consists of three phases: an inhalation, a forced exhalation against a closed glottis, and a violent release of air from the lungs following opening of the glottis, usually accompanied by a distinctive sound and removal of the irritant. The reflexive or involuntary cough may be impossible to completely abolish, but the slight tickle that temporarily spells relief can be, with training of the autonomic nervous system or dilation of the respiratory tree, eliminated. There are

The Good Doctor

cough receptors under the respiratory mucosa, which stimulates the parasympathetic nervous system. But, if it can be cancelled out by the opposing sympathetic system, the cough will be subdued. There may be other mechanisms as noted below that we as humans can willfully do that would work.

My recommendation, as I did myself, is to inhale a rub-on of an aromatic herb on the back of the nondominant hand when I felt a cough in the making. (In that way one can use the dominant crease in the elbow into which to cough if not suppressed by this maneuver.) There are many essential oils that one could use such as Angelica root, Beth Root, Cacao, Cajeput Oil, Colt's Foot, Elderberry, Fennel Seed, Horehound, Mullein, Mustard, Red Poppy Flowers, Thyme, Valerian root, Wild Cherry Bark, and the Mints (peppermint and spearmint). I suggest the most economical that one does enjoy. For me it was spearmint.

Deep breathing activates the parasympathetic nervous system, which induces the relaxation/bronchodilation response. My "HIGH FIVE" breathing exercise works as a natural tranquilizer for the nervous system. I breathed in for a count of five, held it in my lungs for another five count, then exhaled slowly with my tongue on the roof of my mouth and the lips pursed for the last tally of five.

If related to the vital vibrations of the essential oil or the dynamics of airflow with the Bernoulli Principle is a moot point. If one exhales slowly through a small aperture, then the more the tube expands, the less the tissue touches itself. The closer the walls of the bronchioles are to each other, the more likely it is to "self touch" and to stimulate their receptors and cause the cough reflex. After a week of desperate endeavors, I have successfully "cured" my difficulty with extinguishing of the stimulus, the urge, and consummation of the cough!

THE NODES HAVE IT: THE JOHN CASTRO STORY

WHAT WILL THEY CALL IT?

I actually have two findings named after me. The first, "Block's Thumbs," are a sign of the patient's dominant side. The nail on the thumb of the dominant side is wider and more squared off than the thumb on the nondominant side.

This is significant because it's critical to quickly determine a patient's dominant side in the moments following a stroke. It is known that the right brain controls the left side and vice versa. So if a patient has had left-brain damage, the right side would be affected. However, if the person were left-brain dominant, more of their speech and cognitive function would be compromised and the prognosis (which is the eventual outlook for recovery) would be worse than if the patient were left-side dominant.

After my article appeared in the *New England Journal of Medicine* it went viral...at least what we considered "viral" before the Internet came along. It became a question on Hollywood Squares (a television game show) and an entry in *Reader's Digest*. But I knew I'd really hit it big when my second grade daughter brought home her Weekly Reader with a mention of Block's Thumbs in it!

The eponym named after me is "Block's Blotches," which are the small red bruises found on the skin of the arms, particularly the back of the hands. I wrote an article on my findings in the *New England Journal of Medicine* in 1970.

What I had discovered is that people with these blotches tend to be older than their stated age, drink too much alcohol, suffer from diabetes, and/or they took cortisone. Of more interest to me was that all the folks I saw with these red blotches tended to be much more susceptible to infection.

The Good Doctor

I found that these blotches were caused when there was trauma to a small blood vessel resulting in red blood cells leaking into the surrounding subcutaneous tissue. This would initially cause a red bloodstain, which would immediately cause the white blood cells, whose duty it is to eat up red blood cells, to go to work. Within these cells the red hemoglobin is converted to another pigment, which is brown (bilirubin), then greenish (biliverden) when it metabolized to another pigment.

Looking at the tissue with the naked eye, the spot in the skin undergoes a color change reflecting the change occurring in the blood; the blotches begin to look more like a bruise, becoming black and blue before changing again to a brownish-yellow color several days later. Gradually the blotches fade away as the white blood cells and their pigmentary load find their way back to the spleen and other tissues in order for the iron to be reclaimed by the body and used again.

However, sometimes the blotches can remain for weeks if the white cells are slow to do their work. Of particular medical interest to me was that in the groups mentioned above, old age, too much alcohol, diabetes, and cortisone, all these conditions cause the white blood cells to function poorly.

The end result is that these cells, called macrophages, don't do their job of eating bacteria properly. Therefore, the red blotches indicate that the person could be much more susceptible than average to get bacterial infections. Likewise, the bigger these blotches are and the longer they stay, the more vulnerable the patient is to significant bacterial infections.

These two findings have helped me not only diagnose but help determine an eventual outcome in many of my patients over the last forty years that I've been using these tools.

THE NODES HAVE IT: THE JOHN CASTRO STORY

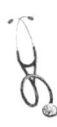

In John's case, the results of the much-awaited blood tests came the next day, and they were telling. The tests were positive, confirming my suspicions of the day before. John indeed had bacterial endocarditis. I knew I had to act fast. I called Dawn to see if she could bring John in. His condition was very serious, and it wasn't just a simple case of the flu. John was, in fact, dying. I told her I needed to see them both as soon as they could get to the office. Dawn said that she wasn't sure she could even get John out of bed and down the stairs to the car given his balance issues, which had even gotten worse over the last few days. I told her to try her best and to let me know if she couldn't get him to the car. I was willing to make a house call if necessary.

Dawn was able to get her very sick husband to the car and they made it to my office. I met them in the parking lot so they wouldn't have to go through the effort of coming into the office to see me. I saw John briefly before telling them to get to the ER. John had a serious infection in his body and time was of the essence.

Dawn got John to the ER and after assessing his situation, the doctors there admitted him and immediately began to treat him with antibiotics. Finally, John's body started to respond and fight back against the infection. He bounced back in good form and was able to be released from the hospital a couple of days later.

But the success was short-lived. Within a few short days, John was sick again and back in the hospital. The medical team tried the antibiotics again, but this time, the infection was relentless. John suffered a couple of minor strokes while in the hospital this time.

The Good Doctor

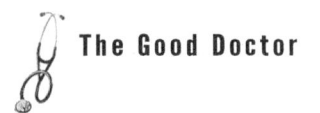

The doctors diagnosed John with an acute case of endocarditis, which is an inflammation of the inner layer of the heart, known as the endocardium. The infection had settled in John's aortic valve and the doctors now determined that the damage was beyond repair. They would have to go in and replace his heart valve.

John was shocked. How did he go from being a normal healthy man to a guy near death? John's friends and family felt the same way. How could this have happened so quickly?

John steeled himself for the coming ordeal of invasive surgery to replace the heart valve. He knew it would be a long process of recovery but was ready for anything that would help him to feel better.

John fought hard and was able to survive the surgeries. But he lost a lot of blood in the process. He had to get several transfusions, making him fragile. His condition slowly began to improve. The new valve was working just as it was supposed to and his body was responding well.

That was a very close call. I'm glad I saw John when I did. When I first saw the results of John's blood test, I knew I couldn't treat him directly. I was convinced he needed to get to the ER immediately, and I'm glad they followed my advice. John and Dawn's faith in my advice ended up saving John's life.

REBUILDING FROM THE INSIDE

But after surviving the surgery, John needed lots of help rebuilding his strength, and that's something I knew I could help with. I was able to recommend several nutritional supplements

THE NODES HAVE IT: THE JOHN CASTRO STORY

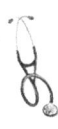

that would help John recover his strength. These supplements, along with a few other dietary alternatives, would get John on the road to recovery just that much quicker.

Today, John is fully recovered. He takes a blood thinner to help ease any strain on the new heart valve, and he continues to take the supplements I initially recommended. John counts himself very fortunate. Not many people get that close to death and recover as successfully as John did. He knows it could have been so much worse.

I've asked John about what made my approach different from all those other doctors he saw while in the hospital. He told me something very interesting. He said that while the physicians in the hospital did a wonderful job and were able to save his life, he always felt like a patient. He felt like he was one of many—a line item on a very long list. But with me, John said he felt much more like a real person with real health issues. John said that he felt like I treated him like a friend.

That blesses my heart. That's intentional. To my mind, the person who sits in front of me is the only patient I'm treating. I just can't ignore the care and compassion that seems to get pulled out of me with every new patient. I connect with them on a very deep level because of their pain and fear. I can't help but get deeply involved with everyone I treat. That's why I'm willing to make house calls. That's why I'm willing to go to the parking lot to meet a patient to keep them from having to get out of the car. That's why, as in John's case, when a patient doesn't have insurance, I'm going to do everything I can to help them find less expensive options.

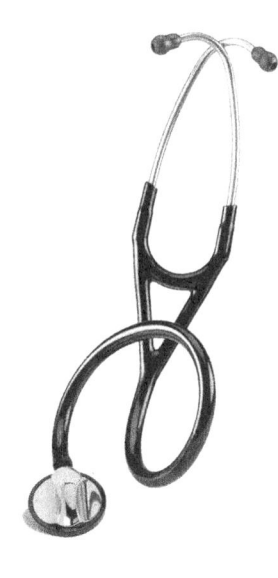

CHAPTER SEVENTEEN:
SERIOUS SINUSES: CAROL'S STORY

I'd love to think that I was on my game every single day. It'd be nice to believe that each day was made up of victories and successes. But just like everyone else, I have my off days from time to time. There have been plenty of times when I haven't done everything right, times when I've missed the most obvious of symptoms or failed to listen closely to what the patient was desperately trying to tell me.

I've suffered from attention deficit disorder for many years. My ability to focus has never been a natural gift, but rather a skill I've been able to develop over many years of very hard work. My nature is to only glance and skim and then move on to the next problem or patient. In fact, I will often tell patients to give me short and concise answers to my questions because

The Good Doctor

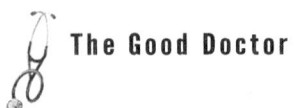

I know the tendency of my mind to wander during long and drawn-out replies.

When Carol first came to see me, I was unintentionally ignoring her primary concerns. She'd been waiting to see me for over five hours, and her hypoglycemic condition had made her aloof and cranky. I was in a similar mood myself. It was after 6:00 in the evening on a day when I'd seen (once again) way too many patients and had more lined up to see when I was through with her.

CAROL'S MISERY

Carol had grown up in Tulsa and graduated from Will Rogers High School. Following school she began a long-time career in the oil industry and married her husband Austin, who was beginning a military career about the same time.

Everything was looking up for Carol. Her job was going well, and her marriage had started off on the right foot. The world was beginning to open up for her. But there was a problem. Carol had suffered from the time she was ten years old from terrible sinus infections. For years, she had struggled through her day with flu-like symptoms. She was constantly exhausted, but too miserable to sleep. Her sinuses would swing like a pendulum, back and forth between being stopped up so she couldn't breathe and running to the point where she couldn't stop the flow.

Carol had made the arduous circuit through the Tulsa area Ear, Nose, and Throat (ENT) specialists. She'd even visited a variety of allergy clinics in search of what might be causing her terrible sinus problems.

SERIOUS SINUSES: CAROL'S STORY

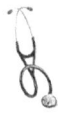

The doctors would routinely prescribe antibiotics, which would improve her condition, but only temporarily. While she was taking her medication, her symptoms would decrease but the minute she ran out of pills, the infection would rage again causing the debilitating symptoms to return with a vengeance.

Of course, growing up in Tulsa only exacerbated her condition. Tulsa is one of the worst cities for those suffering from allergies. Both Oklahoma City and Little Rock are among the top ten worst cities for allergy sufferers according to the Asthma and Allergy Foundation. Tulsa sits in the breezeway between those two allergy hot spots.

Carol had always had to struggle to maintain her attendance in high school, and now she had to muscle herself out of bed just to make it through her days at work. She was determined to be the best employee she could be, but her symptoms of exhaustion and blocked sinuses made it a tough task indeed.

She continued to make the effort to see whatever new allergist or ENT who happened to be recommended at the time. Many of these doctors were quite good, and several came very highly recommended. Carol always tried to expect the best with each new appointment. But even the best of these doctors had no answers for her.

After a thorough exam, one of the doctors returned to the exam room with the results of the latest battery of tests. His shoulders fell as he looked at Carol and admitted that he couldn't help her; he had no answers for her condition.

In desperation, all he could offer her was the recommendation that she move to a different climate, one not so tough on her allergies. He made a few suggestions and offered her the best of luck as she left the office.

The Good Doctor

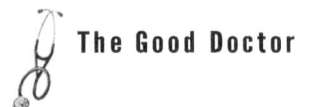

NO GOOD CHOICES

Carol found herself with no good choices. She could remain in Tulsa, but that would mean a life of continual suffering. She could move to another city, but there were no guarantees there either. She and her husband could go through the effort of moving away from their home only to find out the climate of the new city was no help at all. She'd still be sick, but now she'd be far away from her family and friends. Her much-needed support group would be too far away to help her through the difficult times.

Carol and Austin put a brave face on things and reluctantly left their home and family in Tulsa and moved to Arizona in an attempt to distance themselves from the things that were making Carol so miserable. They made their way west to a new home and what they hoped would be a relief for Carol's battle with the sinus infection.

But the symptoms followed her to Arizona. Like a nightmare, the exhaustion, the pain, the sleepless nights, the headaches, and blocked sinuses never eased up. Not even a bit. Carol continued to see doctors in Arizona, but they were mystified just like the Oklahoma doctors were. No one had answers. Now, with no relief in sight and homesickness bearing down, Austin and Carol moved back to Tulsa after just three years away.

They arrived back in town and found a new doctor with a new idea. They would operate on Carol's sinuses and see what was going on. Maybe surgery would be the long-lost answer. While they had her opened up, they'd be able to more effectively investigate and deal with the problem directly. Carol was encouraged.

SERIOUS SINUSES: CAROL'S STORY

But after three unsuccessful surgeries Carol finally cried, "ENOUGH"! She had endured decades of doctor visits, pills and shots, an exhausting move to Arizona, and now painful and invasive surgeries, all to no avail. The ordeal of trying to get well was becoming more exhausting and frustrating than dealing with the illness. She finally relented and accepted the fact that she would just have to live with this condition for the rest of her life. It obviously wasn't what she wanted, but she figured it was her only real option.

UNTIL ONE DAY

Until one day...

Just like Crystal, one day Carol heard me on the radio. For years, whatever city or town I found myself in, I would broadcast a weekly radio show in the local market. I'd go on air for about an hour and talk about the new things I was learning and my beliefs about practicing medicine. I found that not only did this weekly radio conversation help build my practice, it also helped answer questions many people had about their own personal approach to health.

Carol resonated with the program and became a regular listener. She heard me talking about my integrative approach to healing—combining natural and traditional methods. She perked up and immediately began to take notice. She was convinced that all the medications she had been taking had been a double negative for her. Not only had the meds not worked, but also many of the side effects she'd had to deal with were far worse than the sinus infections. She knew that couldn't be good for her.

The Good Doctor

From listening to me on the radio, she knew I knew what I was talking about. Gradually she began to think I was someone who could help her with her life-long struggle. She could tell from listening that I not only understood the science, but I knew the human body as well. And more importantly, I understood how everything worked together. She called my office and made an appointment to see me as quickly as she could.

A BAD START

But things didn't start off well.

I had moved my office from Coffeyville, Kansas, to Tulsa and my practice had exploded. In addition to the overwhelming response from new Tulsa-area patients, many of my Coffeyville patients continued to see me, willing to make the long ninety-mile trek south.

Because of the crush of patients in the new Tulsa office, Carol had to wait over five hours for her first visit to see me. It's never fun to have to wait long but to have to wait that long after making an appointment is unforgivable. I'm surprised she waited. But if you were to speak with Carol today, she'll tell you that at the time she was so desperate she was willing to do whatever it took.

What's amazing is that Carol was dealing with another health issue in addition to the sinus infection. She also suffered from hypoglycemia. As those with hypoglycemia know, unless you eat every three to four hours you'll begin to suffer from blurry vision, a rapid heartbeat, extreme fatigue, headaches, and more. As you can imagine, Carol was not a happy camper by the time I walked into the consultation room!

SERIOUS SINUSES: CAROL'S STORY

I must've made a good impression upon entering the room because she didn't immediately chew me out for having to wait so long. Many days, I won't wear my doctor's "uniform." I won't wear a white lab coat, and I won't have my stethoscope around my neck. In many cases, this can confuse a patient a little. It's as if I'm not a real doctor. I come across completely different from their expectation. I've found that sometimes that can be a good thing.

The reason I don't always wear those things is that I want to immediately put the patient at ease. From the time I come into the consultation room, I work hard to knock down any barriers that might hinder open and honest sharing together. I want the patients to be completely open and frank with me about their health issues. I don't want to be untouchable, just the opposite! I want to be completely approachable, and over the years I've found that sometimes the "uniform" can be intimidating to some patients.

Carol was willing to wait the long five hours and put up with the eccentricities of my busy practice only because she was so desperate for answers. After hearing me on the radio, she had pinned all her hopes on me. I began our visit by asking her a series of questions not having much at all to do with her sinus issues. I was looking at the much bigger picture of what was going on with her overall health. My mistake was never keying into the fact that Carol was suffering from a very serious sinus infection. She was frustrated with me, but that's just how distracted I was that day. I didn't even notice.

I didn't even end up seeing Carol until almost 6:00 in the evening, and it was quitting time for me. Carol was dealing with her hypoglycemia, and I was dealing with my ADD. It's a wonder we got anything accomplished at all on that very first

The Good Doctor

visit. She was fading fast, needing something to eat, and I had a hard time keeping my focus on the task at hand. But we made it through...barely. Carol was so desperate for answers that she actually agreed to a follow-up visit.

Carol continued to visit me about once a month, and we would take up where we left off. When she'd come for her appointment, she'd either see my colleague, Lindsey Berksen, or me. But things weren't progressing like Carol needed them to. She was still suffering terribly from the sinus infection, and she needed help—help I wasn't giving her. She knew she was going to have to do something drastic in order to rattle my cage enough to get my attention. I'm ashamed today to think that she felt like it was up to her to get me to focus on what she knew her problem was.

Carol was irrigating her sinuses every morning and evening like she'd been doing for decades. She'd done it so much, in fact, that the habit was much like brushing her teeth. The process involved mixing a saline solution and placing it in a squeeze bottle or a large syringe. She would tip her head to the side at a forty-five-degree angle so her lower nostril was over the sink. She would continue to breathe through her mouth while squeezing the solution into her upper nostril. The solution would pass through her sinuses and drain out of her lower nostril and into the sink.

But this time she altered the process. This time she was very careful to catch the nasty drainage in a container. She poured the ugly mixture into a Ziploc bag and sealing it carefully, brought it to her next appointment. While she waited on me to enter the room, she couldn't help but check her purse to make sure the bag wasn't leaking!

SERIOUS SINUSES: CAROL'S STORY

AN UNWANTED GIFT

I walked into the consultation room and sat down on my roller stool just like I always did. I rolled over close to her and asked how she was doing and after some small talk, she couldn't stand it anymore. She was ready to spring her trap! She reached into her purse, grabbed the bag, and tossed it on the table between us.

You can imagine my surprise! In almost fifty years of practicing medicine, nothing like this had ever happened to me before. I was used to having the upper hand in these patient visits, but she had reversed the roles. I didn't know what to say or how to respond. I just sat there staring at that vile plastic bag. She pointed to the bag full of her nasty drainage and cried out, "Dr. Block! That's the stuff in my head! That's what is making me so sick! I need your help! I'm sorry, but I don't know any other way to get your attention!"

I looked at the bag and then back up to Carol, then back down to the bag. I might get distracted from time to time, but Carol had grabbed my attention. Clearly, this was a woman in pain. For the first time, I turned my complete focus on her painful sinus condition. I knew then that I had to attack this head on. Carol needed answers; she had waited long enough.

I began to ask about her lifetime of dealing with this condition. I asked which doctors she'd seen and what they'd recommended. With Lindsey's help, we dove into her history with all the energy we could muster. We both realized that I had a lot of lost time to make up for. I asked Carol about the pills and the shots, the surgeries and allergy clinics.

The Good Doctor

For the first time in months, I was asking her questions she felt were relevant to her condition. The answers poured out. She couldn't get the words out fast enough. My assistant, serving as a scribe, was taking furious notes on her tablet.

We found out about the lifetime of antibiotics and the fact that they had never actually worked, at least not for long. It didn't take long for me to figure out what the problem was. All those years the doctors were treating what they thought was a viral infection. But that's where they missed it. If the infection were viral, the antibiotics would've brought Carol relief.

IT MUST BE FUNGAL

So, if the infection wasn't viral, it must be fungal. I immediately put Carol on an antifungal medication that she could take in pill form. She left my office that day with a bottle full of new pills and good reason to believe that her condition would improve. For the first time in years, she felt a small glimmer of hope begin to peek out from behind the dark clouds.

From the very first dose, Carol began to feel better. Within a few days, the sinus issues had almost disappeared.

But she wasn't out of the woods yet. There was a problem.

Carol's sinuses were clearing up and healing for the first time since she was ten years old. But she was feeling terrible. In fact, she seemed sicker now than she'd been in years, sick to the point that she couldn't even get out of bed.

She came to see me and we immediately began the investigation process to find the problem. We were thrilled that the antifungal pills were working on her sinuses but, of course, she couldn't live life feeling sick like this. We buckled down to find the answers.

After some research, we found that the antifungal medication in pill form was actually causing her blood sugar to drop. She was suffering from all those familiar hypoglycemia symptoms...but this time it was the antifungal pills that were causing the problem. Worse than just being unable to get out of bed, Carol was so weak she was almost in a coma.

I immediately recommended that Carol go to a local "compounding" pharmacy. This is a pharmacy that resembles more the apothecary shops of our past than the modern Walgreen's or CVS on the corner. Their volume of customers and prescriptions makes this level of customized service prohibitive.

A compounding pharmacy takes the time to combine medications into compounds, customizing the medications specifically for each patient. After ample and careful input from us, they were able to put the antifungal medications into a nasal spray form. This allowed her body the benefit of the antifungal meds without them becoming absorbed into her bloodstream.

Since Carol has started taking the new medication, her life has completely changed. She takes the nasal spray morning and evening and for the first time since she was ten years old, Carol has her life back. Now that we have the sinus problem solved, we've been able to focus on Carol's other issues.

INSOMNIA

Carol struggled with insomnia for many years. No doubt her initial problem began as a side effect of the many medications

The Good Doctor

she was taking. But the problem lingered, and she was unable to sustain consistent sleep, never allowing her body to get the complete rest she needed. It's been proven that several serious health issues can be improved simply by getting more sleep. Lack of sleep can cause accidents, reduce sex drive, inhibit cognitive tasks (the ability to learn), cause depression and much more. Loss of sleep certainly wasn't doing Carol any favors. It was making the other things she was suffering from much worse.

Through the years, the doctors had prescribed Valium to help Carol sleep better, but the Valium wasn't working. She was still losing sleep. When I learned of Carol's insomnia, I started her on progesterone. Now she sleeps all night and has noticed that, with more sleep, she is better able to ward off the nagging infections that continue to attack her body.

FINDING THE RIGHT PACE

I continued to see Carol about once a month to make sure we stayed on track with her ongoing healing process. One day Carol got very sick just a couple of days before a scheduled appointment to see me. She was feeling terrible, so badly in fact, that she almost called to cancel her appointment.

She came in the office and I could immediately tell that something was wrong. Like everyone who comes for an appointment, one of the very first things we did that day was to check her blood pressure. Her systolic blood pressure (the first number) was over 200! The systolic number is a measurement of the blood pressure in the arteries when the heart beats, that is, when the heart muscle contracts. The diastolic number,

SERIOUS SINUSES: CAROL'S STORY

the second one, measures the pressure in the arteries when the heart is at rest, between beats.

We quickly performed an EKG test. The EKG revealed that her heart was beating erratically and skipping beats frequently. In typical situations like this a doctor of traditional methods would likely put her on a pacemaker. But as you know by now, I'm not a traditional physician!

I suggested a compound of minerals including magnesium and potassium to be taken every day. Since Carol has begun this regimen, her blood pressure and heart rate have gradually been brought under control. Carol is ecstatic. She's in a much better place now, and all without the invasion and life adjustment that installing a pacemaker would have brought.

Most recently, we found blood in Carol's stool. At any age it is suspicious of an intestinal malignancy. Although the Colon Century Test returned, showing a "low chance of having cancer," I treat the patient, not the test. So we ordered a colonoscopy that showed a small "abnormal area" on the right colon and within a week Carol was scheduled for surgery. During the procedure, the surgeon found a small cancer and removed it. In just two days she was able to return home and soon felt as good as new.

Carol says, "Dr. Block's knowledge and understanding of the human body, the science and how it all works together, has made a believer out of me. His curiosity and quest for knowledge didn't stop when he finished medical school. I love the fact that he's never limited his treatments to the more traditional methods. He's open to whatever is going to get me well. He even expects me to be a student of what's going on in my

The Good Doctor

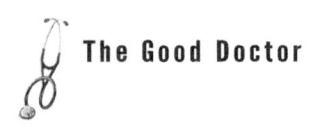

body! I never leave his office without a stack of papers and a book or two with the assignment: READ!"

That's been a tenet of mine for many years. I know that I'm not the one in charge of a person's health and healing. That's the purview of the patient. I'm simply there as an advisor, a guide, a consultant, and I hope, a trusted friend. Thanks to the invaluable input from my colleague, Lindsey Berksen, we were able to help Carol on her road to a much healthier life.

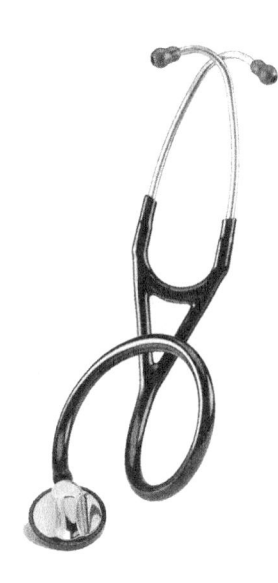

CHAPTER EIGHTEEN:
MY SPIRITUAL JOURNEY

Looking back over my life, one thing has always been very clear to me. Things that seem to fall naturally into place for some people have never come as naturally for me. Many of the things that I've achieved or experienced in my lifetime have come through a lot of trial and error. I'll have to say that in many cases, I haven't been the first on board or the quickest learner in the class, but when I do get a handle on something, I've got it for life. I've never been a tentative person. It might take me a while before I'm ready to take the step, but when I've made the decision to step out, it's all the way and with both feet. Once I'm in, I'm all in.

This has been true of my medical career and true of my spiritual journey as well.

In 1993, I made the conversion from Judaism to Christianity, and in many ways, it also marks the beginning of

The Good Doctor

my transition from Physician to Minister. The dictionary defines "minister," as "one who gives service, care, or aid...." By that definition, I guess I've been a minister since I started my medical practice, but I know several times over the years when I've turned to a Higher Power for guidance in helping my patients. To me, it's always been a spiritual journey. As you can imagine, there's much more to this story. In order to understand completely, you have to grasp the unique relationship I have with my son-in-law, Dean McQuillan, and his unique walk of faith. Dean was instrumental in guiding me along this path.

MEETING DEAN

In 1979, I was dating my wonderful wife-to-be, Brunie. At the same time, her daughter was dating a young man by the name of Dean McQuillan. Dean is a gregarious and open man with a quick smile and a ready handshake. When I first met Dean, he was a successful car salesman in Kansas City. His career was on the rise, and he was just starting to reap the benefits of his hard work.

In much the same way, I was living the life of a successful doctor. While it's true that early in my career money wasn't a motivator, I'll admit that over the years in practice I had grown accustomed to the many trappings of my success. By that time I had fully bought into the idea that the things I owned were an accurate measure of my success, the more I owned, the more successful I was. In fact, I had adopted the attitude that the one who dies with the most toys wins. Dean and I had that attitude in common. He was a success in his career, and I was a success in mine; and both of us had our share of toys.

MY SPIRITUAL JOURNEY

We'd get together often, living only a short distance from one another. When we'd meet, we'd share a drink and talk about where we were in our respective journeys. We'd compare notes on our most recent purchasing conquest. I can't say that we were competitive, but I can say we always kept one eye on our scoreboard to see who was ahead! As we shared life together, I felt like our relationship was deepening. Our friendship was growing and it was a blessing to grow so close to a new member of the family.

THE WINDS OF CHANGE

But there were changes in the wind. Dean and Dorlisa, Brunie's daughter, began attending a large church in Kansas City. Over the months, I could see their priorities starting to change. The accumulation of wealth and the things that accompany that wealth was no longer top on Dean's priority list. I could feel a shift beginning to occur in our relationship. It was subtle at first, but it was to become much more pronounced later. We no longer shared the same goals or passions. It felt like Dean was drifting further and further away with each visit. Sometimes it seemed that, except for being family, we had very little else in common. By 1981, Dean and Dorlisa had both given their lives to the Lord. It was clear now that everything had changed.

Dean's interest in spiritual things was a lightning bolt out of a clear blue sky. He was raised in a home by parents with no interest in spiritual things at all. Dean would say his parents didn't have an ounce of godliness in them, no awareness and no acknowledgment. God had no place in Dean's home growing

The Good Doctor

up, not in his family or his life. When the time finally came, Dean didn't just get saved. He got radically saved!

I still remember listening to him share with me about his newfound faith on one of our first visits after his conversion. Dean couldn't help blasting me with his new beliefs. He'd pound me with both barrels! Dean would tell me frequently, "Jerry, I know you're Jewish! But I believe in the greatest Jew who ever walked the planet! I want you to believe in Him too!"

A NEW LEVEL OF SPIRITUALITY

However, instead of attracting me, Dean's spiritual zeal and passion drove me away. I had never known someone who had had an experience like Dean's. Our times together became very awkward for me. Despite my efforts to reach out, I had trouble connecting with the "new" Dean. I couldn't understand how he could become so focused on his spiritual life and his new faith in God. Dean was unlike other religious people I knew. Strict rules and rituals from the outside just didn't motivate him. He was driven by a deep passion that bubbled up from the inside.

Given my Jewish upbringing, I knew I believed in the same God as Dean. But my spiritual beliefs were all about actions and activity, following the Jewish calendar. To me, to be a faithful Jew was to follow a list of things faithful Jews did. It wasn't about changing the person you were on the inside. It was all about following the list of rules and rituals on the outside. I had been faithful all my life to observe the Jewish traditions and rituals, careful to do the right thing at the right time, and I was very religious in the way I clung to those beliefs. But I would never assume that these actions would change me.

MY SPIRITUAL JOURNEY

Dean was talking to me about an entirely different level of spirituality. He was talking about an actual relationship with God. Clearly, something radical had happened in Dean's life and he had changed down to his very core. There was a dramatic shift in his priorities. His life was no longer about pursuing things or the accumulation of wealth; it was about finding treasure in his relationships with others.

These beliefs began to affect more than just Dean's priorities. They were changing his behavior. The Dean I used to know didn't exist anymore. He no longer cared to share a drink with me, choosing instead to abstain from alcohol entirely. His language was no longer peppered with "colorful" words like it was before. Dean was indeed changing. It was as if he had become a different person, and this was making a profound impact on me. While I didn't know it at the time, these were the initial seeds of Christianity being planted deep in my soul.

Dean's new faith seemed to be driving him to do things that lacked even common sense, at least from my perspective. Dean had quit his very successful career at the auto dealership in order to return to college and get his Theology degree. While I am a huge proponent of education, this move made no sense to me. Why give up such a promising career and throw it away on something like religion? It baffled me at the time.

But Dean was no longer listening to me. He had new influences in his life. He was now driven to succeed in an entirely different arena with new rules and new definitions of success I knew nothing about.

With a new degree in Theology, Dean was ready to step into a whole new way of life. He proudly announced that he was accepting his church's call to a new work in Dillon, Montana.

The Good Doctor

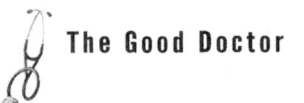

Brunie and I were very concerned. Okay, we thought, change your views, change your priorities, and even change your career. But move over 1,200 miles away from your home and your family? That's crazy!

TRADING ROLEX FOR TIMEX

It wasn't until Dean's farewell message to his home congregation that he won me over. Because we are a very close family, we made the decision to go to the final church service, even though the move confounded us. I'm glad we went. At the service, I was finally able to grasp Dean's new motivations. While I didn't accept them for myself yet, Dean's spiritual journey was beginning to make some sense to me.

In Dean's message, he told the congregation that he was trading his Rolex watch for a Timex watch. In that simple statement, he was able to encapsulate his shift in priorities in a way that I could understand. Ever since I first met him, Dean had worn a Rolex. It was one of his symbols of success. He wore it proudly, as he should have. But once he received his call to Dillon, he knew the Rolex on his wrist would send the wrong message to the folks he was going to minister to. He selflessly gave the watch to his mentor, the man who had led him to Christ and had continued to be a tremendous influence in his life. He had the back of the expensive watch inscribed, "To my Paul, from your Timothy." Dean traded his Rolex for a Timex.

I was at once stunned and convinced. Dean's conversion was real; there was no denying that. His words impacted me profoundly. This wasn't a flash in the pan whim. This wasn't a decision you make one day only to walk away from it on another. I still wasn't ready to convert, but I could now see how genuine Dean and Dorlisa's new faith was and the lengths they were willing to go to follow their new path.

DEAN'S MOVE TO DILLON

Over the coming months, Brunie and I made the trek westward to Montana frequently to pay visits to Dean and Dorlisa. I watched as Dean's church began to grow. I figured that Dean would be a success at whatever he put his mind to. He's sharp, has a great sense of humor, and is very personable. I knew he'd do well in this new church. But I was not prepared for the rapid growth I saw in each return trip to Dillon.

Dean's church, known as Grace Baptist Church, started in a living room but quickly outgrew that space. They moved into a classroom of the local college. When they outgrew that space, they moved into the auditorium of the school. Soon they were busting at the seams of the auditorium and needing to build a building of their own.

THE PASSOVER LAMB WAS THE KEY

Meanwhile, God was building something in my own heart. Back in Coffeyville, Kansas, I had been invited to a Passover service and meal by a patient and friend of mine who also happened to be the pastor of the local Lutheran church. I had participated and even helped to lead Passover services many

The Good Doctor

times. I just assumed that this would be another Passover service along the traditional Jewish lines I was used to. I had no idea this particular service was sponsored by an organization called Jews for Jesus! This service was different in a very significant way for me. In the message, the sacrificial Passover lamb was compared to Jesus Christ...the Lamb of God.

That was it! For me, it was the missing link. I finally understood what Dean had desperately tried to get me to understand through countless conversations over the years. That night, the ball dropped into place and it all finally made sense to me. This new revelation did much more than just open my ears. It opened my heart to the things God was trying to tell me.

I was excited to tell Dean what had been revealed to me at the Passover meal. When I got him on the phone, I practically shouted, "Why didn't you ever tell me about those things? I never realized that Jesus was a symbol of the Passover lamb! I get it now!" Not being Jewish, Dean had trouble getting it. The way you talk to a Jew about spiritual matters is much different than the way you would speak to a nonbeliever.

The fact was, I already believed in God. I knew God and prayed to Him twice every day! I thought that's all I needed. I didn't believe that I needed an intermediary until I heard about Jesus within the context of Passover. Of course, I was familiar with the Old Testament, but turning to the New Testament gave me a whole new appreciation for scripture and our need for Jesus and His saving grace. I read about the Apostle Paul, who was known as Saul before his conversion on the road to Damascus. Paul's life was completely changed because of Jesus Christ. That got my attention.

MY SPIRITUAL JOURNEY

SPIRITUAL ANSWERS ON A LEGAL PAD

While I was closer than ever, I wasn't ready yet to surrender to Jesus. I needed more answers. I needed to connect the dots between what I'd heard in the Passover service and the scriptures from the Bible that backed it all up. I knew Dean could help. His preaching style had always been to shore up all of his points with a solid scriptural foundation. So while I had him on the phone I asked Dean if he and Dorlisa could help. They promised to write me with all the scriptures I would need.

Dean and Dorlisa got a legal pad and sat down that very night and wrote out scriptures that would help me fill in the missing pieces of information. They laid out in a very logical and orderly way the steps one takes to accept Jesus Christ as the Lord along with specific scriptures for every step. Then, at the very end of the five or six pages of notes, they added one more little tidbit of information, just to make sure I read the whole letter. In the very last paragraph they inserted the sentence, "Oh yeah, by the way, Dorlisa's pregnant!"

When I got the letter in the mail, I sat down with Brunie and walked through each of those bullet points. The scriptures opened up to us as we looked up every verse. Questions we'd been holding on to for years fell by the wayside. We were convinced that God was speaking to us through that letter and through every scripture we read. Then to read at the end that Dorlisa was pregnant was just icing on the top. We gratefully...and finally both asked Jesus Christ to be our Messiah, to be our Savior as we asked Him to dwell in us and be our Lord.

It was Easter Sunday in 1993, and we couldn't wait to call Dean and Dorlisa to give them the news. We knew that Easter would be an exhausting day at the church, so we mustered all

The Good Doctor

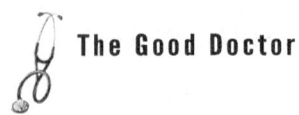

our patience and waited, giving them time to get home from the Sunday services and lunch. Through many tears, we explained that we'd finally and completely given our hearts to Jesus. We all wept together, so grateful for what the Lord had done in our lives. Then, almost as an afterthought, we congratulated them on the coming new life. God had given us new life and even marked the event with a new life for Dean and Dorlisa.

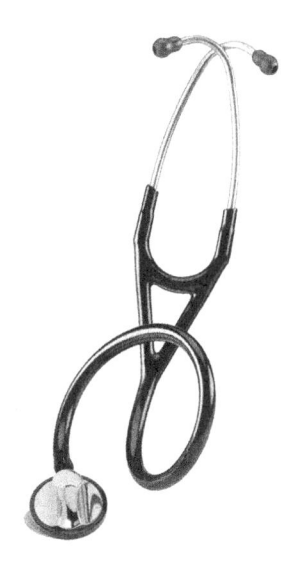

CHAPTER NINETEEN:
SPIRITUAL LESSONS LEARNED

Though I was saved and had asked Jesus to come into my heart to be my Lord and Savior, I still had difficulty coming to grips with a couple of foundational Christian beliefs.

The first was baptism. The concept of baptism was a difficult one for me to understand. Dean tried over and over to explain it to me, but I wasn't able to grasp its significance. Even though the practice is described in the Bible, I just couldn't get why it was necessary. I resisted Dean's attempts to get me under water.

In the summer of 1995, we planned a guy's trip to Glacier National Park. I was going to get to travel with my boys...my son and my sons-in-law. We had a wonderful time and saw some beautiful country. We had the opportunity to spend lots of quality time together. We got to relax and talk about the

The Good Doctor

deeper things in life. Of course, Dean continued to encourage me at every turn to get baptized.

STRIKING A DEAL

It was on a hike up Little Chief Mountain, just south of the beautiful St. Mary's Lake that the conversation finally came to a head. I challenged Dean and made him a deal. I told him that if he'd hike with me all the way to the summit of the mountain, I'd get baptized. Dean's competitive spirit kicked in. We leaned into the effort and made our way up the steep switchback trail.

After a few hours of steady climbing, it became obvious that we wouldn't have enough daylight to make it to the top of the mountain. Dean is an athlete and was in tremendous shape. He was moving up the trail like a mountain goat, and I was doing my best just to keep up. I suggested that, to make better time, we forget the switchbacks and just head straight up the mountain. Dean nodded his assent and left the trail, climbing in earnest straight up the steep mountainside through the scree at first, then the snow and ice. His determination and youthfulness took over. He was leaving me further and further behind.

The altitude and steep icy trail finally took its toll on me. I was struggling and couldn't keep up his pace. I thought I would die trying to get to the top of that mountain. I was ready to concede and called up to him, "Enough! I can't keep up! You win! I'll get baptized!" I surrendered that day to Dean…but I also surrendered to the Lord. We gave up the quest for the summit and headed back down the mountain to the car. I was already trying to imagine what the baptismal service was going

SPIRITUAL LESSONS LEARNED

to be like in Dean's church. I'll admit, confessing my devotion to Christ and being dunked under water in front of several hundred strangers was not very appealing.

BAPTISM BY ICE WATER

Dean had other ideas. Now that I'd agreed to baptism there was no way he was going to wait for us to get back to Dillon.

We drove down the road from the mountain, but Dean turned the van in a direction we hadn't been before. He drove right up to the shore of St. Mary's Lake and stopped. He turned to me and said, "Are you ready?"

"Ready for what?" I questioned.

"Ready for your baptism!"

"What? Here? You're crazy! I thought you were supposed to be baptized by fire, not by freezing water!"

He smiled at me and said, "There's no time like the present!" He got out of the van and came around to get me. I was torn. I really did want to be baptized, but this was happening pretty quickly. I began to balk but Dean picked me up out of the car and carried me down to the water's edge. He looked at me and smiled as he put me down. We held hands and walked into the water together.

Standing almost hip-deep in the water we turned and faced the shore and the loving faces of my boys. Dean put his arm around me to steady me and encouraged me to place my arms across my chest and hold my nose.

The Good Doctor

As Dean said, "In the name of the Father, the Son, and the Holy Ghost" we bent backward together and I went under water. Needless to say, the temperature of the water nearly took my breath away!

Right there in the beautiful, clear (and freezing!) waters of St. Mary's Lake, in the shadow of Little Chief Mountain, and surrounded by my boys...I was baptized. In the same way I was overcome by the frigid water that day, I was overwhelmed by the love of my boys, my family, my relationship with the God of my father but also the new loving relationship with my Messiah. I came up out of the water and Dean gave me a big bear hug, followed by hugs from all the guys. I walked out of St. Mary's Lake that day a new man. Since that day, Dean and I have reminded one another that while he ministers to people's spiritual lives, I minister to their physical ones.

UNDERSTANDING THE TITHE

The other Christian concept I had trouble with was tithing, which, looking back, you think I'd understand because tithing was first introduced by God to the Hebrews. It was a Jewish practice long before it was a Christian one.

We were on vacation one time with Dean, Dorlisa, and their kids. We were in Hawaii; Dean was watching football in his hotel room, but I wanted to play in the surf. I had plans to go boogie boarding with my grandson Ryan. I burst into Dean's room to get Ryan, and while I was waiting for him to get ready, I began to pepper Dean with questions about tithing. I just couldn't understand why God would want me to give back to

SPIRITUAL LESSONS LEARNED

Him 10 percent of everything I earned. Of course, I ignored the fact that Dean was trying to watch the game. I had questions that needed answers!

Dean patiently told me that God honored the tithe and that it was all His anyway. We are not owners of the things we have, only stewards. He said that God blesses us so that we can be a blessing to others. I heard what he was saying but still had trouble with the concept. I worked hard for the things I had. The last thing I wanted to do was start giving things away. Before leaving the room, Dean offhandedly said, "You might as well give to God. He's going to get it eventually anyway!"

Before leaving on vacation that year, I had purchased a beautiful diamond ring. In the same way that Dean's Rolex made a statement about his career, I felt my ring did the same thing. It was obviously expensive, and I thought it showed the world how successful I was as a doctor. I was so proud of the ring; I wore it everywhere I went. I even chose to wear it to the beach that day with my grandson.

Ryan and I had such fun at the beach that day boogie boarding and playing in the surf. It wasn't until after an hour or so that I suddenly realized my ring was missing! I was having so much fun I didn't even realize that the ring must've come off in the surf. We searched in vain for that ring for a long time before finally giving up and admitting the obvious; the ring was gone for good.

I was angry with myself. It was foolish to wear that ring in the water. On the way back to the room, I remembered Dean's words, "You might as well give to the Lord. He's going to get it eventually anyway!" Then I became angry with God! He took my ring!

The Good Doctor

I stormed up to Dean's room and burst in yelling, "You S.O.B.!" I still had a ways to go in learning to curb my temper and my language! Dean said, "What are you talking about?"

"I lost my ring in the water! God stole it from me!"

God certainly moves in mysterious ways. He taught me a lesson about giving that day that has stayed with me ever since. From that day forward, I understood that God blesses me, not so I can simply have more things. God blesses me so that I can be a blessing to others.

It just so happened that the ring was a kind of test. God was preparing me to give to Him and His work in a much bigger and more profound way.

INVITED TO DO BIG THINGS FOR GOD

Dean's church was busting at the seams. To make matters worse, they were meeting on the fourth floor of an old building on the college campus in town, an old building with no elevator! That meant each week they'd have to lug sound equipment and other odds and ends up all those stairs for Sunday services. Then after the services, take them all back down and store them away for another week. To say this was getting old would be an understatement.

Dean had a big vision to build a brand-new church complex with not only a building for church services, but also a parsonage for him and his family and a full sports complex. Dean was an athlete and came to the Lord through the sports programs of his Kansas City church. His vision was to duplicate that program in Dillon.

SPIRITUAL LESSONS LEARNED

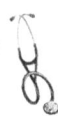

He'd found an ideal piece of property about a mile north of Dillon. It was an old twenty-acre sheep ranch that still had a couple of homes on it. Dean had heard that the property might be up for sale, so he grabbed one of his deacons and paid a visit to the landowner.

The lady confirmed that the land had been for sale but that it had recently sold. A horse rancher who was a surgeon from New York had offered to pay cash. Although the sale hadn't gone through yet, it was practically a done deal.

Dejected, Dean and the deacon started for the door when, like Columbo from the old television series, he stopped in his tracks, turned and asked her, "I have one more question. If the buyer backs out and chooses not to buy, could we have the first shot at it?"

She said, "Well, it's a done deal. But yeah, if the deal falls through, you'll have the first shot."

Dean said, "That's all I ask."

Six weeks later Dean got the call. The deal had fallen through.

The lady told him that he could buy the land for $250,000.00 and not a penny less. She'd carry the note, but she'd need $35,000.00 down. Now Dean was in a bind. He'd put himself in a position to buy the land, but the church had no money! He knew he could manage the financing—he'd subdivide the land and sell off the portion with the two houses that the church didn't need—but the plan hinged on the down payment. Where in the world was Dean going to quickly find $35,000.00?

That's when Dean called me.

The Good Doctor

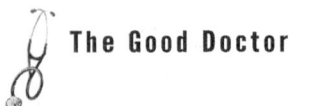

When I answered, the first thing Dean said to me was, "Jerry, how would you like to be a part of something really cool for God?"

"What is it?" I asked, my curiosity piqued.

He told me the whole story. He said, "I need to borrow $35,000.00 from you. I'll pay you back within a year along with interest."

At that moment, I remembered all the things God had been teaching me about being generous. Saddling Dean with interest didn't seem right to me and I told him so. I offered him the money interest-free and told him to pay me back whenever he could.

Miraculously the church was able to pay me back in full within six months! And this is from a church of only five hundred people in town of only 5,000 with an average salary at the time of just $19,000.00! Not to mention that the town of Dillon is made up of mostly Mormons!

But the miracles didn't stop there. The church was able to raise over half a million dollars to build the beautiful facility debt-free. Today that church reaches out to much more than just the town of Dillon. Its influence stretches throughout the county and beyond to surrounding towns. They've even planted a sister church an hour away, in the city of Butte.

To think that God allowed me to be a part of His plan for Dillon is humbling. So many lives have been changed because of a single obedient, generous act. God had blessed me so that I could be a blessing to the folks of that community and beyond. I've seen the lives of folks who have come to me for treatment dramatically changed. But to be able to impact the lives of those I have never met is incredibly fulfilling. God taught me an important lesson: never cling to the things that belong to God anyway.

A WHOLISTIC APPROACH

King David wrote a psalm I love,

What is man that you are mindful of him, and a son of man that you care for him? Yet you have made him little less than a god, crowned him with glory and honor. You have given him rule over the works of your hands, put all things at his feet: All sheep and oxen, even the beasts of the field, the birds of the air, the fish of the sea, and whatever swims the paths of the seas. – Psalm 8:5-9 (NABRE).

Some scholars think man is little more than an animal, but there are others who would lift man almost to the position of a god. There are also those who would combine the truths of both and see man as a strange dualism, something of a dichotomy.

There are depths in man that go down almost to hell but there are also heights that can nearly reach heaven. Man is a biological being with a physical body. The Bible states we need more than just the daily bread in order to survive. If we stop here we would see man merely as a human animal.

But we are so much more. The human is much more than the sum of its parts. Because of our prefrontal lobes and the volume of our cerebral hemispheres, we can not only remember the past as we interpret it, but we can also see our future, even though it may never come to pass. The fact that we are multi-dimensional is more than just a simple hypothesis.

The Good Doctor

Humans have conscious and unconscious aspects, rational and irrational features. We are a body/mind being. Not just intellect, but emotion, intuition, and instinct. Our instincts have been honed and fine-tuned over the last million years.

Therefore man has insight, rationality, logic, emotion, hunches, gut feel, creativity, rhythm, and a beautiful sense of harmony that brings all these things together.

People use information gathered from their five senses to guide them and help them interpret their world. However, I believe there are more than just the five senses. I believe there's a sixth "special" sense that's well above our physical perception. There are those who have it and those that just survive. To be in possession of that sixth sense is to become close to perfection, while not having that sense is like most of the human race...just surviving, not really living.

In the days following my acceptance into medical school, I felt that sixth sense. I felt my being becoming whole. What I had longed for for so long had come to pass, and it clicked in me in a very profound way.

Of course, history has proven that I'm far from perfect. My sixth sense has aided me time and time again in my practice, and I truly believe it has helped me to become a better doctor. But perfection is still a long way off. In the end, I'm a mere mortal.

AN INTEGRATED SPIRITUAL JOURNEY

Thinking back over my life, it's no wonder my spiritual journey reflects the integrated approach just like my medical

SPIRITUAL LESSONS LEARNED

journey has. I grew up Jewish and then converted to Christianity. But that's not to say I've thrown out my Jewish beliefs, quite the opposite. I cling to the beliefs, traditions, and rituals now as much as ever. But I'm also a devoted believer in the Christian faith. In fact, as I look across my own deeply personal and individual spiritual landscape, I can see elements of many different faiths, many different paths.

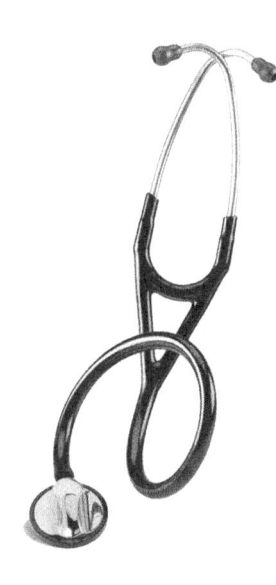

CHAPTER TWENTY:
OUR UNWRITTEN STORY

I've always felt that an abundant life is one of vitality and verve to the very end. However, this is a pretense and not true, especially in today's modern world. Ninety percent of us will end up not dying in peace and dignity. For this reason our story needs not only a good beginning and middle but also a wonderful end.

Life is a nonfiction narrative. Like most stories, this account should not only be meaningful, but also memorable. We humans begin our self-record at about age three when there is some comprehension of meaning and past verbal memories, just like my memory of the closet under the stairs. It's about that time we start writing the tale of our life. We do this by "self-talk."

The Good Doctor

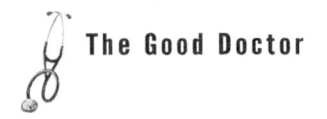

MEMORY ALTERS REALITY

Fundamentally, our memory goes through our emotional filter and we remember our lives differently compared to reality. Because actuality is obscure, our inner speech gives a report of perception and self-deception. Healthy minds rationalize life in its best light so we can live with ourselves knowing that we have done the best anyone can under the circumstances. No one thinks they are boring or average. We would all like to think we're from Garrison Keillor's fictional town of Lake Wobegon, "Where all the women are strong, all the men are good-looking, and all the children are above average."

In the end, it is what people tell themselves happened rather than what happened that becomes their life story. There is a semi-constant internal monolog a person has with oneself on a conscious, semiconscious, and dream level. Thoughts are in the third person, and our activities are observed as in a video or movie.

Children narrate their actions out loud before replacing this mode with the adult equivalent of subvocal articulation. During subvocal articulation, no sound is made but the mouth still moves. Eventually, we inhibit our mouth movements, but the experience of words and pictures is captured in our memory bank as our story is written over time.

The healthy human mind minimizes the negative and painful moments and maximizes the pleasurable, positive ones. A sick mind reflects an event in a painful and adverse mode. Life is the composite of the emotion and the intellect, encompassing the understanding of the world and our role in it. We weed out the things that are not important in our self-dialogue. It also gives the presence of mind needed to make crucial decisions based on experience personally or vicariously. The life story is a series of meaningful happenings with the nonsignificant ones deleted from the visual text. How we seek to spend our time depends on how much time we perceive ourselves to have. When we are healthy and young, we believe we will live forever.

LIVING HAPPILY EVER AFTER DOESN'T JUST HAPPEN

A good story is always one that ends well. That's why the best stories end with "…and they all lived happily ever after." A good story is not just about a collection of the targets we've shot toward or the goals we've achieved. In the beginning chapters of our life story, we view our life as growth and plans for fulfillment. Nurturing, achievement, education, social connections, physical and emotional love are all recorded.

As we mature, security is significant for us and for our loved ones. Toward the end of our story, we focus on what is most meaningful for the soul. Family, a few close friends, and what we have contributed to the world begin to take center stage. As we age, it is the satisfaction of a job well done that counts, not the excitement or the exhalation.

The final chapter of our story must have fulfillment in order to be meaningful. It is not how well someone has lived, but how they finished that is most significant. We want to die in peace, not in discomfort and suffering. The standard answer to the mode of death is to go to bed and "wake up dead"! The fact is, we will be "with the Lord" or in oblivion forever, depending on our beliefs. Most would like to believe the former, but it is not our decision.

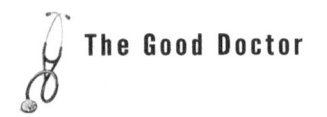

LEAVING A MEANINGFUL LEGACY

Our future is finite. In order to finish well, we must put our personal affairs in order. Not just our Last Will and Testament, but the legacy we leave to our family and others. The most important personal affair we put in order is where and how will we spend our last days.

End of life preferences need to be discussed with family and health providers so we can die in peace, in full control of our situation. The medicalization of taking care of this aspect of life can turn our blissful tale to woe. Times have changed. No longer do we die in the privacy of our bedroom and family but in nursing homes; many times our discomfort made even worse in the intensive care unit bed with tubes in every orifice.

But there is now. Right now. We've all been blessed with the gift of today. I'm reminded of the overused Latin phrase, "Carpe Diem," or "Seize the Day." I've been very fortunate in my years of practice to be able to work with thousands of patients who are doing just that. They don't know what the future holds, but they have today and they are committed to making the most of it. We can all learn from their example.

NO LONGER THE SCARED LITTLE BOY

I hope I've learned and am making the most of every single day I have on this planet. I'm no longer the three-year-old little boy trapped in the closet under the stairs. And while that experience was traumatic for me, it's molded into my life characteristics that have made me the good doctor I am today. I can trace my insatiable desire to help my patients back to those dark experiences I had as a little boy. I'm more compassionate, more attentive, and more sympathetic because I've felt the sting of fear, abandonment, and betrayal. Truly, what the enemy meant for harm, God has turned to good in my life and for that I am grateful.

Throughout my life I've been blessed to have been surrounded by a wonderful family and great physicians, like Drs. Erber and Kahn and Drs. Jeghers and Worley and so many more. Doctors who were dedicated to the same cause as I have committed my life to, to see to the care and well-being of those who have entrusted that care to me. And it's to those patients, folks like John and Kaye, Crystal and Rose, Carol and John and thousands of others who have taught me the most valuable lesson of all; I don't know everything, far from it. While I'm grateful to have had some answers along the way, I know I have so much more to learn. My journey isn't over. The goal of being a good doctor is never fully achieved. I pray that I'll never lose the desire to learn, to discover, and to push the edges of my own ignorance. To me, that's what being a good doctor is all about.

I want to challenge you today, on the last paragraph of this book to seize each moment life brings. Live life to the very fullest. Grab every opportunity you can to find meaning and significance. Take the time to realize that you are writing the last chapter of your story right now…today. Write well, my friend, while you are in command of the story. You are the only person for which it is meaningful. This is the only activity in

The Good Doctor

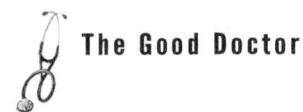

which we will see ourselves living happily ever after. Make your presence in your world meaningful!

CONTACT

For more information, to send a comment, or to purchase books, please contact:

docblockbook@gmail.com